How Toxic
Are YOU?

How Toxic Are YOU?

"Is your suffering tied to toxins inside you? Discover what people just like you have to say about improving the quality of their lives using the ideas in this book. You deserve to have the best life possible today and every day. Enjoy the book and don't hesitate to contact me with your own personal success story."

- Dr. James H. Martin

The Solution for Body Pollution

DR. JAMES MARTIN

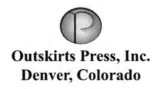

Outskirts Press, Inc.
Denver, Colorado

How Toxic Are You?
The Solution For Body Pollution

Outskirts Press, Inc.
http://www.outskirtspress.com

ISBN: 978-1-4327-5138-8

Outskirts Press and the "OP" logo are trademarks belonging to Outskirts Press, Inc.

PRINTED IN THE UNITED STATES OF AMERICA

DISCLAIMER

The information contained in this book is based upon the research and personal and professional experiences of the author. It is not intended as a substitute for consulting with your physician or other healthcare provider. Any attempt to diagnose and treat an illness should be done under the direction of a healthcare professional.

The publisher does not advocate the use of any particular health-care protocol but believes this information in this book should be available to the public. The publisher and author are not responsible for any adverse effects of consequences resulting from the use of the suggestions, preparations, or procedures discussed in this book. Should the reader have any questions concerning the appropriate-ness of any procedures or preparation mentioned, the author and the publisher strongly suggest consulting a professional healthcare advisor.

ACKNOWLEDGEMENTS

To my loving wife Christine, who shares in my values of education and integrity and fills our home with love and encouragement for our family to aspire to their dreams.

To my daughter Ashley, who shares my vision in her work in alternative medicine, my stepsons Nick and James for their support and my parents for always believing in me.

To all the members of The Natural Health Association, your drive and passion to reach for wellness through natural methods is commendable. You have been an inspiration for me everyday, every week, and every year of my life.

A special salute goes to those of you who have shared your personal health 'Success Stories' with the readers of this book.

Know that your words may have lit another's path along the road to wellness.

With gratitude I thank each of you who gave your help in getting this book out to the masses…Jeanie Glass, Jeff Ryan, Linda Scheerle, RN, and my entire staff whose belief in this mission makes me hugely proud.

I continue to discover…….

"Together we CAN make a difference!"

FOREWORD

"Dr. Martin has made it an integral role of his 30 year professional career to educate others about the body's natural ability to do
battle against the onslaught of noxious and harmful substances that
modern society indiscriminately tosses into our environment. Now
he has encapsulated his findings in an easy to read and informative
book that will certainly open your eyes to just what is waiting for
you inside and outside your front door. However, rather than leav-
ing you confused and befuddled Dr. Martin provides suggestions for
fighting back, what to avoid, simple products that you can make, and
tips to improve your lifestyle. He leaves few stones unturned. This is
both an educational and enjoyable read that will certainly return an
investment to the health of the reader and their family."

-Mark Scheutzow, MD, PhD, NMD, FAAIM

TABLE OF CONTENTS

How to Slow Down the Aging Clock

INTRODUCTION

The slow poisoning of the population of the United States yields huge profits for mainstream medicine. Treating symptoms with drugs makes billions for the pharmaceutical companies. Costly diagnostic testing, invasive procedures and surgeries keep hospitals, laboratories and medical supply companies in the black. Insurance companies pass these high costs onto policyholders, the ones who can still afford health insurance coverage.

Has spending more on traditional healthcare than any other country in the world made us *healthier* as a nation? The statistics show we are far behind most other industrialized nations, and even *lead the world* in the highest incidence of breast cancer.

With soaring health insurance costs and drug costs, shouldn't we be getting better quality care as a result? What happened to the 'War on Cancer'? Why have cases of cancer, heart disease and diabetes become *more prevalent* in the last few decades than *less frequent?*

As long as mainstream medical researchers and practitioners *continue to ignore the environmental and dietary causes of degenerative disease,* the grim health statistics will continue to worsen, and more people will suffer from earlier onsets of ill health.

Who's to blame? By allowing manufacturing industries, agribusiness and the military to pollute our air, water and soil with chemical toxins and heavy metals, we've opened the door for trouble. Factory farming has provided us with hormone-fed animals to enhance their growth artificially. Ever-increasing pesticide use on food crops, lawns and golf courses has disrupted our neurological and hormonal systems, and those of birds and amphibians. Our insatiable demand for processed foods and plastic (a petroleum derivative) has resulted in a daily intake of solvents, synthetic dyes, and endocrine-disrupting chemicals entering our bodies. With over 70,000 new man-made chemicals created and put into use since the Industrial Revolution, *what have we done to our bodies?* Consider also the pressure to vaccinate our children with numerous mutated viruses, in serums known to contain aluminum, formaldehyde, mercury and other toxins. And shall we *really* trust the multi-national food makers who splice our food particles with DNA from animals, insects, chemicals and viruses?

We pay the high price everyday. These chemical toxins in our lives and in our food have compromised our good health to such a degree we now see children with hardening of the arteries, high blood pressure, higher rates of juvenile-onset diabetes, autism, and other developmental disorders. Adults are succumbing to more neurological diseases at earlier ages, such as Alzheimer's, Parkinson's, MS, ALS (Lou Gehrig's disease), depression and anxiety disorders.

We wonder how much school violence, street crime, domestic violence and child abuse has been caused by toxins in the brain? How many marriages and families fall apart because nutritional deficiencies and toxicity played a major part?

Where *can* we go to escape the toxic pollution? To a faraway island? Poisons have filled our air, soil and water worldwide. Even in the Antarctic, scientists had to drill 50 feet into the ice to find ice which was free of DDT, a pesticide banned in the 1970's. Even polar bears reveal DDT stored in their fat, living far away from factories and auto exhaust. So there *is* no 'safe' place to live and be isolated from the onslaught of toxins. Besides that, I happen to *enjoy* living and working in the USA; I would imagine many of you do, also.

Is there an 'escape' from the perils of body pollution? The recent 'Green Revolution' is beginning to raise awareness somewhat. Consumers are finally starting to choose less-toxic cleaning products, personal care products, and healthier food. Organic food availability is becoming more widespread. While these are 'baby steps' in the right direction for Americans, *the build-up of brain and body pollution will not be undone by suddenly switching to fragrance-free detergent or buying free-range eggs.* Our immune systems are under siege by rampant bacteria and viruses; but our bodies often fail the fight against these invaders because of the enormous load of chemicals and metals we need to detoxify.

Our built-in pathways to process-out toxins and poisons are clogged, overloaded and bearing a burden the human body was not designed to handle. Possibly in another 10,000 years (if we survive as a species) we will adapt our inner filtration systems to handle these 70,000 new chemicals without suffering harm. That concept of adaptation offers some hope for future generations; but our current population is in the midst of a nationwide health crisis. These cries for help in the form of disease, birth defects and a myriad of symptoms *are not being adequately addressed by mainstream medicine.*

The design plan of the human body is not to be faulted; I'm actually surprised more people are not dropping dead everyday from the poisons in our food, air, water, prescription and over-the-counter drugs. Our bodies have an incredible built-in potential to heal; *but when we take drugs to cover-up symptoms—we merely shut off the broken pathway and ignore the hidden causes of the problem.*

Some toxins don't even cause obvious symptoms as they build up to dangerous levels. Lead, for example, may manifest only as a lowered I.Q. in a child, yet causing bigger problems as time passes. Fluoride, widespread in public water supplies and toothpastes, may cause fatigue, lethargy or brittle bones yet go undetected for one's entire lifetime. Common cold viruses and dental bacteria often lie dormant while slowly infecting the heart, leading to heart disease.

In view of this eye-opening information, I have made it my life's work to enlighten others about the power we each have to rid our bodies of the toxic burdens that are killing us.

When we identify and remove the overload of environmental chemicals, metals, molds, yeast, fungi, parasites, biotoxins, mycoplasmas and mycotoxins, (chemicals produced by fungi) then *the body has a chance to begin to repair and rebuild the cells, glands and organs under attack by these offenders.*

As we enhance the function of body systems with specific targeted nutritional formulas, we can speed up the healing process dramatically. *This strategy works with the body, and does not add to the toxic load, as with synthetic chemical drugs.*

As an alternative practitioner for over 30 years, I have personally seen many people (both young and old) recover from grim diagnoses, and prognoses, assigned to them by their medical personnel. Although *no* health practitioner can honestly promise you a 'cure' for any ailment or disease, you *can* arm yourself with knowledge, new information and pursue health choices that you might not have been aware of until you read this book.

Your body was designed to be healthy, to live a fully active life well into old age, free from chronic disease and pain. By setting the stage for *healing to happen,* you will be amazed at your body's inner recovery power! Only *you* hold the power to take responsibility for feeling good and being well. In the pages that follow I offer insight, information and hope to those of you who truly want to feel good and are ready to take action to protect your health…..*before* a health crisis limits your choices or ends your life.

Wishing each of you will take the smartest steps on your journey to shining health,

Dr. James H. Martin

CHAPTER 1

LIFE-CHANGING EXPERIENCES

Challenges and Triumphs

The main reason for this chapter is to share with you what people have experienced using our procedures and protocols at the Nutrition Wellness Center. It is to give you some actual opinions regarding the effects toxins have and what the possibilities are when toxins are eliminated. Due to limited space I tried to include a variety but limited number of individual's experiences. These were not paid testimonials but actual reports from people who followed our program. I hope you enjoy and appreciate their experiences.

There is no greater personal or professional honor than knowing I have helped facilitate the restoration of health for the individuals whose true stories are printed in this special chapter. I respect their courage for taking the braver, less-traveled road, which is becoming the preferred choice more and more. We cannot guarantee results; but we *can* give you our 30 years experience in nutrition and detoxification. *We guarantee we will do our best* to help you detoxify and create the best internal environment for optimal healing. All statements regarding health testimonials are the reflection of each individual's experience, and do not constitute medical claims by Nutrition Wellness Center, Natural Health Association or Dr. James Martin. Our approach to health shows you how to support your body's normal ability to detoxify, and to help you achieve and maintain a healthy status. By this equation, we do not intend that toxicity is itself a disease; rather if such toxicity is not addressed, disease may result; and without addressing such toxicity all of the body's normal responses to disease may be less effective than they could be.

It warms my heart when I receive these testimonials and endorsements from people who have experienced our program. However, because the testimonials are from lay people, they express themselves differently and share their experiences in a way that is unlike what a health professional would say. You will notice clients talk in terms of their symptoms and how our program helped heal them. As alternative health professionals our focus is not on the person's symptoms, but rather on the cause of their discomfort. The purpose of nutritional support and detoxification is to promote optimal wellness and NOT for the treatment of any disease or health condition. However, our clients focus their comments on their symptoms which, as you read them, may mislead you into thinking our program could cure whatever ails you. This is not the message we're trying to impart. We at the Nutrition Wellness Center and the Natural Health Association of Dr. James H. Martin claim that we will detoxify your body which will in turn increase your feeling of well-being. In fact, in order to better inform you of the results you can expect with our program, we have reviewed our client's beginning toxicity levels in August 2008, and found that four to six weeks later 99% of those people had a decrease in total body burden (toxins). Of that group, the average overall decrease in toxins was 79%. It was this decrease in total body burdens that increased the well-being of our clients, and while their testimonials talk in terms of symptoms disappearing, it was really the detoxification of their bodies that gave them a feeling of relief.

"For three and a half to four years I had daily headaches. I missed a lot of school and never did anything with friends. I had to quit volleyball and basketball. I tried lots of prescribed headache medications. I had CT scan done, I had acupuncture, and chiropractic . . . they didn't help at all.

"We heard about Dr. Martin through a friend who knows Linda, a Nutritional Case Manager and registered nurse who works with Dr. Martin at Nutrition Wellness Center. She told us about Linda's success, so we spoke with Linda, and then came to Nutrition Wellness Center.

"Since coming to Dr. Martin, the kind of severe daily headaches I was getting are completely gone. Also my energy has improved. Everyone at my school and my family has noticed the positive change. And also the people my Mom works with have noticed—she's my high school principal.

"The Nutrition Wellness Center is a hidden treasure, because there are a lot of people who don't know there's an alternative to medications, or who don't yet have an open mind."

—Whitney and Valerie
Bradenton, Florida

"Dr. Martin and the Nutrition Wellness Center offer a unique, comprehensive, and integrative approach to health. My massage therapist first suggested I come to Dr. Martin because I was suffering with migraines. I also had multiple fibroids, ovarian cysts, and a complex ovarian mass in my left ovary region. I had occasional spotting as a result, insomnia, and anxiety. My thyroid gland and metabolism were off as well. My MDs prescribed birth control pills and a sleep medication called Ambien, which caused weight gain and lethargy. They also prescribed Lexapro for the anxiety, which made me feel dopey.

"After several months on Dr. Martin's program, the cysts have shrunk dramatically (documented my Mayo Clinic ultrasound studies). I sleep much better without needing prescribed drugs and their unpleasant side effects. I have not had a migraine in a while now. I will absolutely recommend Dr. Martin to others."

—Julie

Sarasota, Florida

"I came to Nutrition Wellness Center because of having migraine headaches for over 20 years. I've had headaches for as long as I can remember. When I got a migraine, I couldn't function. I had to go to sleep in a dark room. I missed my children's functions.

"I tried taking the prescribed drug called Imitrex. I tried drinking more water, in case they were from dehydration. I tried stress reduction techniques. Nothing helped. Sleep and time passing were the only things that helped.

"I heard about Nutrition Wellness Center though my family. Three of my family members came to Dr. Martin.

"Since beginning the program, I haven't had a headache for a month. I definitely have more energy and I've lost 15 unwanted pounds. My husband has noticed and thinks I look great. I can stay up later at night; and I have more energy. Nutrition Wellness Center is awesome! I will recommend to others."

—Jill

Apollo Beach, Florida

"For several years now I have been trying to make lifestyle changes that would add to my quality of life. Yes, I've made some changes—but spending a week at the Nutrition Wellness Center has given me the courage, and the desire, to make a real transformational change in my life. Each of you, in your own special way, provided such wonderful lessons to be learned, encouragement to change, and nurturing to endure. Your knowledge is phenomenal, your commitment to healthy living was evident, and your path is correct. I feel very blessed to now be a part of the Martin Movement! Bill (husband) too appreciates all you have done for him—his quality of life has improved—to the gym, walking the dog— he will be a lifetime devotee!

"So thanks to each of you to the part you played. Keep doing the great work you are doing, and take great pride in your successes—you are giving people the gift of life!"

—Jan and Bill

Durham, North Carolina

"I had water retention—I definitely notice it is better now. I definitely have more energy and I can sleep better. My gums are not bleeding at all now, and they had been bleeding often for 55 years.

"My gingivitis disappeared completely. I had it for 55 years. Ankle swelling improved greatly. Fatigue—condition improved greatly, the energy increased and I can sleep well without waking up in the night. Weight loss—I lost about eight pounds without dieting. Left sacroiliac joint pain disappeared by itself. In the past six months I had about six chiropractic adjustments; it had improved for a few days, but always returned. After the treatments at Dr. Martin's clinic the pain disappeared without any chiropractic adjustment and had not returned since January (four months). Cholesterol: My medical doctor told me my cholesterol had decreased from 277 to 170 in the last test; he could hardly believe that it was done without pharmaceutical drugs. Three and a half months ago, when I first told him about these cleanses he did not comment, but I could tell by his demeanor he thought not very much of it. On my April 22nd visit he was surprised."

P.S. "The freckles (or age spots) on my hands are fading."

—Aelita

Belleair, Florida

"When I'd wake up in the morning my hands and ankles would be stiff, and my lower back, too. Now my lower back feels like it did 20 years ago. I am so excited! I am so committed to this—it blows me away.

"I tried all these other kinds of diets and Vitamin B12 just to get some energy . . . I would have a little energy and then be tired again in three hours. I was so tired and I was depressed. I didn't want to go to work. I just joined Shapes (Fitness Center) and I am working out. I know I can do it now.

I have recommended Nutrition Wellness Center to others . . . two friends have already come in. I'm telling everyone I know about it now."

—Denise

Sarasota, Florida

"For four years I had bladder leakage, and had to wear pads. After three weeks on the supplements the leakage has nearly stopped, no need for the pads anymore. I feel a lot better; I'm not bloated now. I used to doze off as soon as I'd sit down; people used to laugh at me. Now I don't do that and I'm sleeping better at night. I used to stay awake much of the night. When I'm driving I'm more alert now.

"I can get up from sitting on the floor without grabbing on to anything. My friends are amazed . . . they can't believe the good shape I'm in. I belong to a gym. I'm 80 years young . . . I don't feel 80; and I don't dress like I'm 80!"

—Orma

Brantford, Ontario, Canada

CHAPTER 2

THE WAKE-UP CALL

How Did We Get SO Sick As a Nation?

Is It Really All *That* Bad?

It seems that Americans are more concerned with their health than ever before. We watch what we eat, we exercise, and we drink plenty of water. The healthcare industry has become one of our biggest industries as people line up to try the newest and latest in wellness and exercise products and services.

We *want* to be healthy. We really do.

So why do we continue to get sicker? Why is there a rise in diseases like cancer, thyroid deficiency, obesity, ADD, and ADHD? Why are autoimmune diseases on the rise and why are we more fatigued than we should be? Why do we suffer from depression, and why do our joints hurt? Why, when we spend so much time and money trying to be healthy?

The answer is simple: *toxins*.

That's right. We are simply exposed to more toxins than we can handle.

The human body is an amazing machine. It is actually designed to discharge toxins from the body by the liver, kidneys, lymphatic, co-lon, lungs, and skin. Unfortunately, it is *not* designed to handle the *amount* of toxins most of us encounter today. As more and more tox-ins accumulate in our system, they place severe stress on these or-gans of elimination. With continued accumulation the organs begin to malfunction, causing a weakening of the immune system. And when that happens, guess what? Your body becomes the perfect host to disease and illness.

But wait a second, you say. I'm a really healthy person! I drink my eight glasses of water every day. I eat the recommended servings of fruits and veggies. I do yoga every day.

Well, that's a good start. Your intentions are excellent. But what if I told you there are toxins in the water you drink? That there are toxins in the food you eat. Heck, there are even toxins in the yoga clothes that you wear! As a matter of fact, *toxins are all around us.* They are in the shampoo and cosmetics we use, in the carpets in our living rooms, and in the gas that we need to run our car. They are in the deodorants we use, in the cakes we bake, and in the dye in our hair.

They are *every*where!

Way back when it used to be easy to make non-toxic choices. Until the turn of the century, most all food could be considered health food. Air pollution and water contamination were rare. The ingredients in everything from our cleaning products to our clothing were natural. Then came the advent of synthetic chemicals. Synthetic chemicals were designed to replace natural ingredients. They were cheaper to use and earned the chemical industry a small fortune. They were produced with such a fury that today the chemical industry is the biggest industry in the world. Billions of pounds of synthetic chemi-cals are produced in America every year, with production doubling every ten years or so.

Many of these synthetic chemicals are *known* to be highly toxic. And still others we don't know much about at all. Yet we breathe them, drink them, and absorb them through our skin.

And we can't handle them. Our bodies *try* to do their job. But the fact is there are too many chemicals to process. So what happens? The levels of toxicity start to build up inside of us. Our body systems start to break down. *We are being poisoned.*

Let's consider the health of our society as a whole. It has just been within the last 50 years or so that "new" diseases like ADHD, chronic fatigue syndrome, and autism have reared their ugly heads and are now affecting large percentages of the population. To make matters worse, people are getting sicker at *younger* ages; the number of babies and children contracting chronic illnesses continues to skyrocket. Degenerative diseases are on the upswing, as are diseases such as cancer, cardiovascular disease, arthritis, asthma, autoimmune diseases, thyroid disease, and diabetes. And how about those non-specific, non-diagnosable issues? We all know someone who suffers from fatigue, drowsiness, headaches, rashes, nausea, joint aches, ringing in the ears, swollen glands, hormonal imbalances, sudden hair loss, overall system degeneration, difficulty concentrating, dizziness, restlessness, or irritability. These issues can be life-altering, and yet often doctors can't pin down *why* we have them. They are not associated with any specific illness. And so we remain undiagnosed. And untreated. And the problems continue unabated.

If you think the medical community as a whole should be in an uproar over this, well . . . they are. Billions of dollars have been spent researching why people are getting sicker. Much of the research focuses on finding a treatment. The result is a new generation of medications designed to *suppress the symptoms*. And while the pharmaceutical companies continue to get rich, our health deteriorates. Why, when we have access to all these new drugs? Because the drugs treat the symptoms, but not the *cause* of the dis-ease. And until we address its *causes*—we'll continue to be sick.

Unless you live in a cave, you've seen those reports on the nightly news linking the toxins in our environment to our decreasing health. Consider the following:

- There are at least 20 studies published in peer reviewed journals showing a relationship between pesticide exposure and the increased risk of cancer in children in the form of brain tumors, leukemia, and lymphomas.

- The National Academy of Sciences estimates that 360,000 children have developmental and neurological disabilities due to toxic exposure.

- The EPA considers 90% of all fungicides, 60% of all herbicides, and 30% of all insecticides to be potential causes of cancer.

- In 1973, the National Cancer Institute found a connection between pesticide exposure and 50% increase in lymphomas in Americans.

- In 2003, the Environmental Working Group extensively checked nine adults and found their bodies contained a total of 167 different chemicals. Their urine or blood had an average of 91 different industrial compounds or pollutants.

- The drinking water of 15 to 23 million Americans is contaminated with pesticides, according to the EPA. Extensive herbicide use accounts for much of this pollution.

- About 90% of municipal water treatment facilities lack the equipment to remove toxic chemicals (or the common drugs) found in the drinking water.

- The USDA found as many as 108 different kinds of pesticides on 22 fruits and vegetables, as many as 37 different chemicals on apples, and 16 pesticides on eight samples of processed baby food. Eighty percent of grains tested in the United States were contaminated with pesticides.

- Red meat, fish, and dairy account for 95% of dioxin exposure. Many Americans have dioxin levels hundreds of times above the acceptable cancer level risk set by the EPA.

- EPA studies of hundreds of Americans show 100% of human fat samples contain styrene, which likewise can cause any number of perplexing symptoms, as well as cancer.

- EPA studies of surgical fat samples of more than 400 Americans showed every single person had stored carcinogens and destroyers of heath—dioxins, PCBs, dichlorobenzene, styrene, and xylene. Any *one* of these alone can cause autoimmune diseases, cancers, and nearly any symptom imaginable.

- Pesticides are so potent a trigger for a multitude of diseases, that they merely give rats one dose of a common organic pesticide to cause Parkinson's!

- Penicillin is a mycotoxin. (a chemical produced by fungus or mold, which causes inflammation and lowered immune response) This fact alone can explain its carcinogenicity.

- Cadmium and lead from industrial and auto exhaust can accumulate in kidneys and cause hypertension.

Wow! And that's just for starters!

In addition to synthetic chemicals, there are other things that are contributing to our chronic illnesses. Things like parasites, bacteria, viruses, and mold. And many of these issues go undiagnosed and untreated. The medical community doesn't know what to look for.

Sure, your symptoms. But the underlying cause of your illness—the parasite, bacteria, virus, or mold—remain in your body. And as long as they remain in your body, you won't be able to enjoy long-term health. The big issue with these bugs in your body is they all produce toxins that add additional stress on your organs and tissues. That's right, fungus, mold, bacteria and parasites contribute to your toxic body burden.

So now that you've heard the bad news, let me give you the *good* news. True, it's impossible to completely avoid environmental toxins. As you'll come to understand in later chapters, they are everywhere. However, you *can* maintain your health and vitality in a toxic world.

You've heard it said before—knowledge is power. You need to take responsibility and learn about the effects of what you are coming into contact with on a daily basis. Armed with the right knowledge, you'll not only be able to avoid illnesses and diseases, you'll be able to live your life in optimal health. And who doesn't want that?

This book is divided into two parts.

- Part I will help you understand the effects toxins have on our health. We'll talk about specific environmental toxins, where they are commonly found, and their effects on the body. We'll learn about symptoms related to the build-up of specific toxins, and how to recognize them. We'll learn how to deal with certain diseases you may already have, as well as ways to avoid chronic diseases in the first place.

- Part II will focus on returning you to optimal health. You'll learn how to maintain health and vitality in a toxic world. We'll cover testing procedure, and talk about the benefits of a specific individualized detoxification program. We'll also learn about nutritional and herbal support, as well as how to avoid toxins in your home.

There are a multitude of reasons why you may have picked up this book. Maybe you suffer from a particular disease and have grown tired of treating the symptoms and want to get to the root of the cause. Or maybe you aren't sick at all, but are disturbed by the increase in diseases and illnesses and want to protect yourself. Whatever your reason for reaching for this book, **I can guarantee when you're finished reading it, you'll be amazed the wealth of information you've learned about toxins.**

I wish you a wonderful journey as you travel the road to wellness. To your good health!

CHAPTER 3

TOXINS EQUAL DIS-EASE

Worse Than Germs and More Invasive

"With studying nutrition and its relation to dis-ease for many years, I was frustrated in not being able to cure my own illnesses completely. Some would not resolve at all despite seeing several practitioners.

"Dr. Martin seems to have found the missing link with his customized program. My liver pain of ten months has gone after six weeks. My digestive problem—so severe that I did not want to eat—is gone. The fog is lifting (I'm able to resume my studies) and unrelenting fatigue is many levels better. I am thrilled with the results so far.

"Not only would I recommend Dr. Martin's program, I think everyone needs his Nutritional Analysis to assess the state of their health—even if they feel fine. If someone doesn't feel well, is symptomatic, I would suggest they run, don't walk, to get the Targeted Nutritional Analysis and to begin the journey back to health."

—Rebecca
Bradenton, Florida

Do me a favor. Next time you are in the shower, pick up your bottle of shampoo and read the label. How many of the ingredients do you actually recognize? In most cases, you'll be assaulted by a mile-long list of incomprehensible chemicals.

And if you are like most people you'll shrug, squeeze a bit of the concoction into your palm, and lather, rinse, and repeat.

All in all, human beings are a pretty trusting bunch. We go about our daily lives assuming that the products we use, the water we drink, the food we eat, and the air we breathe is perfectly safe. After all, if that shampoo was *bad* for us some state or federal government agency—the FDA, for example— would let us know, right? Right?

Maybe not. Consider this. Since World War II, between 75,000 and 80,000 new synthetic chemicals have been released into the environment; *less than half have been tested for potential toxicity to adult humans.* **The average home contains three to 10 gallons of hazardous materials, and 400 synthetic chemicals can be found in the average human body. Of these chemicals, many of them are known carcinogens.**

Another amazing study done by the Environmental Working Group (a team of scientists, engineers, policy experts and lawyers who research and expose threats to health and the environment) measured toxins spread by mothers to babies via the umbilical cord. They found that 287 synthetic chemicals were spread from mom to baby, including perfluorochemicals, flame retardants, pesticides, and the Teflon chemical PFOA.

Almost all of the chemicals found in the umbilical cords have been linked to birth defects, developmental problems, cancer, and brain and nervous system disorders.

The truth is, no one knows *how many* toxic chemicals are floating around in our atmosphere. A widely accepted estimated guess is that there are about 100,000 synthetic chemicals used today, with about 1,000 new chemicals being introduced to consumers each year. What most people don't know is that only a fraction of these have been tested for human safety.

How can this be? Don't certain government laws and regulations protect us against harmful substances?

To really understand how well we are protected, clear your calendar for a day or so and delve into The Toxic Substances Control Act of 1976. For those of you interested in the Cliff Note's version, this act allows chemicals to be sold and used unless they are proven to be a risk, and is constructed in such a way we never really know what chemicals are safe . . . until people or animals begin to get sick. But here's the clincher. **The EPA doesn't perform any tests.** Instead, it uses the research results provided by the actual manufacturers. How accurate is the information? Hmmmmm . . . I wonder!

As if this isn't lax enough, health and safety data has been submitted to the EPA by chemical companies for only about 15 percent of the thousands and thousands of chemicals in use today. What are the effects of the other 85 percent? We don't really know. We can only guess.

The fact is, our government lacks the people and the money to test every single chemical that comes on the market. Let's go back to your shampoo, for example. The guy at the FDA is probably using the same product as you are, and he probably knows as much about the chemical cocktail listed on the label as you do. **You may not know this,** *but the FDA does not review or approve products used in cosmetics.* Considering that the average person is exposed to 126 chemicals per day as a result of personal grooming, about one-third of which have been identified as causing cancer and other major health issues, it's no wonder we don't feel well!

Americans tend to think they have better health than people in other countries. And in 1900, this was true. Even in 1950, the population suffering from long-term, chronic illnesses was only about five percent. Today, according to the Center or National Disease Control, *one-third of all Americans suffer from some sort of chronic or recurrent disease.* **Since 1950 the incidence of cancer has increased 85%.** All of this despite the fact that the United States spends more than $1.3 trillion on health care. **What's it going to take before we realize that money and new drugs *are not* going to cure us?**

Why Our Health System Fails

How do our doctors deal with our toxic overload?

Most doctors are not educated when it comes to toxins and their effects on our bodies. They are trained in traditional medicine, and traditional medicine tells them to treat the symptoms as they arise. The problem is, managing the body with drugs and surgery is not *healing* it. It is not addressing the *cause* of the disease or illness.

Too often, treatment includes antibiotics. Did you know that the annual production of antibiotics adds up to 40 million pounds year? Wow! This includes the antibiotics that doctors prescribe, as well as the antibiotics given to chicken, cattle, and other animals that eventually end up on our plates.

The problem is, antibiotics aren't good for us in the long run. Sure they are absolutely necessary in *some* cases to rid the body of bacteria and cure it of illness. But the overuse of antibiotics has resulted in bacteria that are resistant to drugs. The antibiotics that we take when we don't need to, as well as those that are put in our food supply, destroy the good bacteria in our intestines, which weakens our immune system. And what does this mean? It means that the toxins that enter our bodies do *more* damage!

So there you go. Taken as a whole the scene seems pretty hopeless.

Toxins are everywhere, and it seems like there is no escape. We can't rely on the FDA to keep us safe. We can't rely on the EPA to keep us safe. And we can't rely on the medical community to keep us safe.

So who do we rely on? Ourselves. Education is power. You can continue to stick your head in the sand and be part of this big chemical experiment. Maybe you'll come out of this okay, and maybe you won't. Or, you can be aware. You can know where the toxins are and how to protect yourself against them. You can learn how to reverse the damage already done. Your health is in your hands and your hands alone.

CHAPTER 4

THE THREATS: TOXINS IN OUR WORLD

Sneaky Substances and How to Spot Them

Where do we find toxins? They are everywhere. Let's take a day in the life of an average person.

Hillary Healthybody gets out of her memory foam bed and shrugs off her flame-retardant pajamas. She heads to the bathroom where she splashes some water on her face and brushes her teeth. She hops into her brightly colored yoga clothes, and heads downstairs to grab a cup of decaf and a bowl of low-fat cereal topped with strawberries. She drives her car to the gym, where she spreads her yoga mat on the polished wood floor, and gets ready for an hour of relaxing exercise. When Hillary is done with her class, she takes a shower, shampoos and conditions her hair, puts on her business clothes, and heads off to work.

We should all be so healthy, right? But what you must realize that as healthy as Hillary is trying to be, she's fighting a losing battle. Hillary's mattress and pajamas, both coated in flame retardant material, are emitting formaldehyde gasses. The tap water that she has splashed her face with is full of chlorine and fluoride. Hillary's bright clothing contains dangerous dye chemicals. And so on and so on. Her breakfast, her coffee, her yoga mat, and even the wood floor she places it on all contain toxic synthetic chemicals. She tops off this "healthy" morning by using chemical-laden shampoo and conditioner on her hair. See what I mean? *Toxins are everywhere!*

In the following section I would like to talk about common toxins we all encounter just going about our everyday lives. Let's talk about the toxins in our homes, in our foods, and in our prescription drugs. In addition to alerting you to the presence of these dangerous chemicals, I would also like to show you how you can take some precautions to *avoid* them. While it is impossible, in the world we live in, to reduce exposure to toxins to zero, it is possible to cut down on your exposure. Let's learn how!

Toxins in Your Home

Did you know that the average home contains 2 to 10 gallons of hazardous materials? Yes, I want to tell you that the biggest culprit of toxin exposure is in our own homes. Surprising, but true. Let's take a quick look around.

I know it's hard to believe that something as seemingly innocent as your carpet, tile, furniture, toys, cosmetics, shampoos, soaps, and cleaning products are harming your health. After all, these are things that we use on an everyday basis. However, these items contain two groups of chemicals that are responsible for our increasing health issues:

- Toxic heavy metals and other toxic metals.

- Synthetic and artificial chemicals such as halogens, organophosphates, carbamates, solvents, and plastics and plasticizers.

The fact is, the amount of synthetic chemicals that we encounter in our homes on a daily basis is way more than our bodies can cope with. Let's face it; our bodies' natural detoxification systems are not meant to deal with the chemicals, plastics, and solvents we accumulate. As a matter of fact, the properties of many of the synthetic chemicals found in everyday household items are often impossible for our bodies to process. **So what happens when our bodies** *can't* **neutralize these chemicals? They build up. And what happens when they continue to build up?** *They poison our bodies and cause disease such as cancer, cardiovascular disease, diabetes, obesity, anxiety, depression, ADHD, autoimmune disorders, chronic fatigue, and Alzheimer's, to name just a few of today's most prevalent diseases.*

How about this? In just your carpet, tile, and furniture you can find synthetic chemicals such as toluene, phenol, benzyl chloride, formaldehyde, and xylene. And if you think pesticides are just in your food, think again. You can find a wide array of harmful pesticides in plastics, fabrics, mattresses, wallpaper, air fresheners, carpets, paints, toiletries, waxes, and leather.

Much as I would love to make a list of every toxin you encounter in your home on a daily basis, such as list would be impractical and is beyond the scope of this book. However, if I show you some of the more common chemicals and where you encounter them, I think you'll really begin to appreciate how widespread the contamination really is.

Let's talk about some of the chemicals you encounter in your home, as well as some of the health risks associated with those chemicals. And don't worry—we'll end it all with some good news by showing you how you can detox your home. Yes, it *can* be done!

Metals

I'll bet that you are surprised to find out that a whole host of toxic metals—metals such as mercury, lead, cadmium, and aluminum, are present in a wide array of household items.

Interestingly enough, because many of these metals are naturally occurring, our bodies are designed to neutralize and remove them. So what's the problem? To put it simply, our bodies are being exposed to more metals than we can process. Over time these metals build up in our bodies, and what happens? Our health suffers.

Where do we find these metals? Well, you can find aluminum in the cans you drink your soda or beer out of, as well as in the cooking utensils you use. If anything in your home is electroplated, chances are it contains toxic metals. You can find lead in glass as well as in building materials, roofing, cable covering, and paint, as well as in plumbing.

What are the health problems associated with aluminum? Heart attacks and strokes, blood clots, anemia, Alzheimer's, bone disorders, learning disabilities, mental illness, and speech problems. Not a very cheery laundry list, is it?

And the health problems associated with lead are no better. Of course, unless you live under a rock you are well aware of the developmental problems that lead causes when children are exposed to it. Lead causes loss of IQ in children and thinking issues in adults, as well as anorexia, convulsions, confusion, nausea, paralysis, abdominal pain, anemia, visual disturbances, and vomiting.

Halogens

While halogens are also naturally occurring, there doesn't seem to be any doubt that they exacerbate, and perhaps even cause, many illnesses.

So, what are halogens? Well, in their simple form they are chemicals like chlorine, fluorine, and bromine. However, it is important to note that halogens can be used to make more complex, artificially manufactured synthetic chemicals such as organochlorine, organo-bromine, as well as other organohalogens.

How do we know that halogens are dangerous? Why don't we start by looking at what they've been historically used for. Fluorine, for example, is a gas that was integral to the development of the nuclear bomb during World War II. Chlorine is used as a war gas. And all three above-mentioned halogens—fluorine, chlorine, and bromine—are used in pesticides. Halogens make a great pesticide because they do a good job of *damaging living tissues*. So it just makes sense, doesn't it, that they are difficult for our bodies to break down and are the cause of so many of today's health problems?

Where do we find halogens in our home? We find them in our cleaning solutions and disinfectants, as well as in dyes, gasoline, photograph developing solutions, and in toothpaste. Health problems associated with halogens include cancer, depression, diabetes, high cholesterol, immune system problems, infertility, brain disorders, and behavioral problems.

Organophosphates

Just consider that organophosphates were developed as a nerve gas during World War II. Do you really want to be around these synthetically manufactured chemicals as you go about the daily business in your home? Definitely *not!*

Where do you find organophosphates in your home? Well, if you wear flame-retardant pajamas, you can most likely find them there. You can also find them in the flea treatments you use on your pets, in rubber additives, and in certain wood treatments.

The effects of organophosphates can be short term or long term.

Diseases associated with organophosphates include heart arrhythmias, high cholesterol, cancer, allergies, hormonal problems, thyroid disease, immune system issues, anxiety, depression, and loss of concentration.

Carbamates

What are carbamates? They are another type of synthetic chemical. Thought to be slightly less dangerous than the organophosphates, they affect our metabolism and can result in lethargy and a lower energy level. They can also affect thyroid function.

As you look around your home, you can find carbamates in antimicrobial products, such as hand soaps and surfaces that are treated. You can also find carbamates in cigarettes and cigars (another reason not to smoke!), flea treatments for pets, wood treatments, fungicides, metal chelating agents, mothballs, and synthetic rubber.

Solvents

Solvents are another type of synthetic chemical widely used in home products such as toiletries, food packaging, and floor waxes. Their purpose is usually to dissolve and dilute oil and fats.

Take a good look at the products in your kitchen and bathrooms; chances are they are full of solvents. Solvents can be found in toiletries, shampoos, skin-care products (including those labeled "natural" or "botanical"—pay attention!), detergents, floor waxes, metal foils like those used on the top of cream cheese and yogurt, synthetic rubber, and in polystyrene cups, plates, and packaging.

Remember, I mentioned before that solvents are often used to dissolve or dilute oils and fats. Because of this solubility in fats, they can be tough on the brain. Solvents have been associated with different kinds of brain disorders, including Alzheimer's and memory loss.

Plastics and Plasticizers

Take a look around you, and make note of everything you can see that is made of plastics. Just sitting here in my office, I'm noticing that my computer, modem, printer, and fax are made of plastic. So is the container that holds my pencils, as well as the shelving that contains my files. Even the interior of my coffee cup is plastic!

Bisphenol-A (BPA) and pthalates are the two most common plastic additives, and when you consider the amount of plastic that surrounds us, it's not surprising that these two chemicals are widely accepted to be the two most common contaminants in our world today. Ever wonder about that "new car" smell or other odors that emanate from new plastics? Well, that's evaporated pthalates that you smell—and *inhale.*

Previous studies had found BPA causes precancerous conditions, kidney and developmental problems in animals. But the new research published in the September 17th edition (2008) of the *Journal of the American Medical Association (JAMA)* shows that humans could be walking time bombs of health problems due to "normal" exposures to BPA.

British researcher David Meltzer, M.B., Ph.D., of Peninsula Medical School in Exeter, and colleagues measured the BPA found in the urine of 1,455 adults from the National Health and Nutrition Examination Survey (NHANES) which was gathered in 2003 and 2004. Then they looked at the health status of these people whom the scientists note in the JAMA report are "representative of the adult U.S. population".

The results? Dr. Metzer and his team found that average BPA concentrations, adjusted for age and sex, were higher in those diagnosed with cardiovascular disease (angina, coronary heart disease, or heart attack combined) and diabetes.

Those with the highest BPA concentrations had nearly *3 times the odds of heart disease* and *2.4 times the risk of diabetes* when compared with those with the lowest levels. What's more, higher levels of BPA concentrations were also associated with abnormally elevated levels of three liver enzymes.

The Environmental Working Group recommends we avoid baby formula as much as possible, eat fresh food, not canned food. (canned soups and spaghettis have the highest levels) Also, pay attention to the kind of plastics you use for food or drink. **The plastics that have the most BPA are those made of polycarbonate plastic--they are usually rigid and transparent and used for toddler cups, baby bottles, food storage containers and water bottles. They are frequently marked on the bottom with the letters "PC" and the recycling number 7. Plastics with the recycling numbers 1, 2 and 4 on the bottom are better choices. Glass bottles are better than plastic. Metal bottles may not be free from BPA because many are lined with a plastic coating that contains the chemical. Do not use plastic containers to heat food in the microwave, (if you must microwave at all).**

Some plastics are worse than others. PVC, for example, is loaded with chlorine and dioxins. We already know what chlorine does. Dioxins have been linked to cancer, hormone issues, high blood pressure, weight problems, heart disease, autoimmune disorders, and chronic fatigue.

It's not hard to figure out where the plastics and plasticizers are located in your home. They are in anything that contains an adhesive or glue, carpet backing, cosmetics and toiletries, cleaning solutions, detergents, food packaging, ink, paints, plastic bottles, toys, synthetic leather and vinyl, waterproof clothing, plumbing pipes, and anything that is made out of plastic or rubber.

Toxins on Your Table

By now you have a pretty good idea that everywhere you turn, there's a toxin. Whether you are doing something innocent like washing your hair or cleaning out your drain, chances are you are exposing yourself to dangerous chemicals.

That's bad enough. But how about the fact that we *eat* them? That's right! All of those toxins I mentioned above. We actually ingest them through our food and water. There are toxins on your table, and you need to know it!

Pesticides

These days, pesticides just seem to go with food. As a matter of fact, you have to go to great lengths to buy food that has not been treated with pesticides.

What are pesticides? Quite simply, they prevent food from being infested with bugs. But are we all that different from bugs? While it takes a good amount more to harm us than it does to do away with the pests attracted to our food, consider the amount of pesticides we ingest over a lifetime!

Pesticide Content of Common Foods
(From highest to lowest)

- Strawberries
- Bell Peppers/Spinach
- Cherries
- Peaches
- Cantaloupe

- Celery
- Apples
- Apricots
- Green Beans
- Grapes
- Cucumbers

Consider some of these facts about pesticides:

- Over 4 billion pounds of pesticides are used annually in the United States.

- Current law allows 350 different pesticides to be used on the food we eat.

- Of the roughly 900 pesticide active ingredients registered in the U.S., more than 160 have been classified as known or suspected carcinogens by the EPA.

- One study of 900 adults in a National Health and Nutrition Examination Survey found 98% had a breakdown form of a carcinogenic pesticide, dichlorobenzene, in their urine. About 82% had urine containing breakdown products of chlorpyrifos, organophosphate pesticides like Dursban.

- Another study found 92% of 89 school children had traces of Dursban in their urine.

- The EPA estimates that 74 pesticides, including a number

known to cause cancer, presently contaminate the ground water in 38 states.

- The EPA considers 30% of all pesticides to be potential causes of cancer.

- In 1973, the National Cancer Institute found a connection between pesticide exposure and a 50% increase in lymphomas in Americans.

- It is known that 33% of pesticides are suspect or proven causes of reproductive problems and about 25% are known or suspect causes of genetic damage.

- The drinking water of 15 to 23 million Americans is contaminated with pesticides according to the EPA.

- It is estimated that Americans eat as many as 20 or more pesticide-like chemicals in their meals every day.

- Twenty million children under five years of age eat an average of 8 pesticides a day.

- Red meats, fish, and dairy account for 95% of dioxin exposure. Many Americans have dioxin levels hundreds of times above the acceptable cancer level risk set by the EPA.

- Pesticides are so potent a trigger for a multitude of diseases, they merely give rats one dose of a common organic pesticide to cause Parkinson's!

- There is increasing evidence that human cancer may be caused by the Fusarium mycotoxins. Studies have addressed the relationship between exposure to Fusarium mycotoxins, particularly in corn, and the occurrence of esophageal cancer in humans. (the most prevalent toxins produced by fusarium fungal species are deoxynivalenol (DON) and zearalenone.

Fusarium is a common fungal contaminant of grain)

- A study based on an independent analysis of U.S. baby food products found 16 different pesticides in eight major baby foods.

Indeed, it *is* hard to avoid pesticides. However, we can minimize our risk of contact with and ingestion of toxic chemicals. Making wiser food choices can reduce present and future exposure. But think also about the accumulation of toxins from years and decades *past*. Could these unseen poisons be causing you symptoms now? Could they *already* be paving the road to disease? I believe the answer is undoubtedly *yes*.

Exposure to pesticides can cause a wide variety of illnesses and diseases. Ailments like memory loss, altered personality, irritability, dizziness, difficulty concentrating, headaches, pale skin, wheezing and coughing, liver damage, bowel issues, decreased sex drive, muscle weakness, rashes, kidney damage, abdominal pain, bladder irritation, decreased sperm count, chemical sensitivity, cancer, and hyperactivity in children can all be linked to pesticide exposure.

Pesticides Commonly Found on
Lettuce, Apples, Carrots, Tomatoes, and More:

mevinphos, endosulphan, permethrin, methomyl
methamidophos, chlorpyrifos, dimethoate, dieldrin,
parathion, DCPA, ethion, diazinon, malathion, DDT,
chloropropham, aldicarb, chlordane, diphenylamine,
captan, endosulfan, phosmet.

Metals

How about toxic metals? You wouldn't think you would find those in your food, would you?

Well, think again.

Let's take a typical week-night dinner for a family of four. What's on the menu? How about mercury, lead, arsenic, and cadmium?

Where are all these heavy metals coming from? Well, if you drink or pour your beverages from aluminum cans, you are getting a dose of aluminum. But even if you banish these beverages from your table and make iced tea or drink water instead, you are still getting an unhealthy dose of aluminum. That's right. If you use your tap water, you should know that aluminum is also used as a cleaning agent in water processing plants.

How about the fact that aluminum is also commonly used as a food additive? Hard to believe, but food manufacturers actually put aluminum in their foods—on purpose! Considering that aluminum poisoning can cause such effects as abnormal EEG, Alzheimer's, anemia, blood clots, bone disorders, tremors, heart attacks, learning disabilities, mental issues, speech problems, and stroke, it's not surprising that we don't want aluminum on our table or in our food!

And if you think aluminum is bad, consider mercury. Mercury has been proven to be a very dangerous heavy metal. As a matter of fact, the FDA suggests we now limit the amount and type of fish we eat because of mercury contamination. What is a safe level of mercury? Actually, there isn't one. Consider that a former head of toxicology at the World Health Organization put it this way: "There is no safe level of mercury and no one has actually shown there is a safe level."

Mercury as a food contaminant shows up in largest levels in seafood, particularly fish and shellfish such as shark, swordfish, king mackerel, and tilefish. Before you eat another bite of fish, you should know that exposure and ingestion of mercury can cause long-term neurological and nervous system damage. It accumulates over time! And once it is in your system, it requires specific nutritional/herbal recommendations over several months to remove it.

Other heavy metal contaminants that can be found in fish and shellfish include lead, arsenic, and cadmium.

Metals belong in cars, not bodies!

Additives and Dyes

Take a good look around your grocery store. Have you noticed that there is always a section for "health food?" And doesn't this strike you as odd? I mean, shouldn't all food, by definition, be healthy?

In a nutshell, while we are not all that different from our caveman ancestors, the food we eat has undergone tremendous changes since the time of hunter-gatherers. Food used to be *food*. You plucked it from a vine, dug it up from the ground, or took it from a tree. And that was that.

Today, the foods that make up the majority of our diet are highly processed. And these modern, processed foods are full of synthetic chemicals in the form of additives and dyes. These additives and dyes are used to preserve food, enhance its taste, and improve its appearance. *But while we may be eating prettier, longer-lasting food, we are doing so at quite the price.*

Why do food manufacturers use food additives? Consider these facts:

- Additives preserve the shelf life of foods.

- Additives restore the flavor and texture of foods lost during processing.

- Additives stimulate your appetite, as well as tamper with your body chemistry, so that you *crave* more of the food and *buy* more products.

It's hard to believe, but chemical ingredients are used as emulsifiers, stabilizers, and thickeners in your food. Preservatives like BHA and BHT prevent spoilage. Others are used to give foods better colors, tastes, and appearances. Still other agents are used to control the alkalinity or acidity in certain foods.

Considering that there are $4 billion of these additives sold to the food industry every year—you read it right, $4 billion!—we all want to believe that these additives have been tested and found safe. However, a study done in 2000 by the International Food Information Council found that of the original 200 food dyes used, *110 have been deemed unsafe by the FDA*. (The International Food Information Council, a.k.a. IFIC, is a public relations arm of the food, beverage and agricultural industries)

What kinds of effects do chemical food ingredients have on our health? Many believe that additives and dyes have the ability to alter brain chemistry, causing issues such as ADHD, depression and anxiety, irritability, difficulty concentrating, mood swings, and learning and behavioral disorders.

Additives can cause a whole host of other issues. Consider MSG, a popular flavor enhancer most associate with Chinese food but which can be found in many processed foods on the grocery store shelves. Studies with laboratory animals have shown that MSG stimulates the release of hormones, boosts insulin production, and is linked to weight gain in those who consume it.

And how about those artificial sweeteners? Many people have turned to chemical substances such as aspartame instead of sugar. While people often see this as a health-conscious decision, what is the pay-off? If aspartame and sugar are two evils, then sugar is certainly the lesser of the two. Aspartame has been linked with headaches, mood swings, and is thought to contribute to brain, liver, lung, kidney, and lymphatic cancer. While the many diet and sugar-free products you can find on the market are obvious places to find aspartame, be careful. They can also hide in less obvious products such as vitamins, supplements, and prescription drugs.

Food Dyes and Health Effects	
Red No. 3	Thyroid tumors, chromosomal damage
Red No. 40	Lymphatic tumors
Blue No. 1	Chromosomal damage
Blue No. 2	Brain tumors
Green No. 3	Bladder tumors
Yellow No. 5	Thyroid and lymphatic tumors, allergy
Yellow No. 6	Kidney tumors, chromosomal damage

Toxins in Our Food

Consider these facts when it comes to the toxins we encounter in our food:

- Did you know that several items on your grocery store shelves are contaminated with flame retardant residue? PBDE's can be found in fish, chicken, turkey, pork, and all dairy products. The use of this chemical is so widespread that it is actually leaching into our food supply! We know that this toxin accumulates in the body. What are the long-term effects? We don't know yet, but I'm sure we'll find out.

- The U.S. government signed a treaty that has banned the use of methyl bromide, a gas pesticide, since 2005. However, farmers continue to apply for exemptions and win them. And so methyl bromide is still in our food supply.

- The plastic in your food containers and water bottles leaches into your food and your water. One of the biggest offenders is bisphenol A, (BPA) which is known to disrupt the endocrine system and can affect learning, memory, and mood.

- How are most pesticides introduced to the human body? Through the food people eat. In a nationwide test done by the Centers for Disease Control, the pesticide TCP was found in 93 percent of the test subjects, while DDT was found in 99 percent.

Chlorine, Fluoride, and Our Water Supply:
They Think These Things Are *Good* For Us?

With all of these toxins in our water, it would be nice to assume that at least the water we drink is safe. It is safe, right?

Wrong! By now you know the types of chemicals that can show up in your tap water: everything from pesticides to residues from personal care products, from rocket fuel to heavy metals.

But I want to pay particular attention to two chemicals that are actually put in your tap water on purpose. *I'm talking about chlorine and fluoride.*

Chlorine is used to combat the toxins and pathogens in water that can cause disease. **But did you know that what's put in your water to purify it may be** *causing* **cancer and heart disease?** The French, with their lower cancer rates from consuming resveratrol in red wine, have made red wine famous for its health benefits. There is another side to their low cancer rate that most people don't know— *the French do not drink chlorinated water.* They ozonate their water to purify it. Does this make a difference? Absolutely!

Here's another thing you should know. We don't use chlorinated water because it's *safe*. **We use it because it's** *cheap*. We essentially still pour bleach in our water before we drink it. The long-term effects of chlorinated drinking water have recently been recognized. **According to the U.S. Council on Environmental Quality, "Cancer risk among people drinking chlorinated water is 93% higher than among those whose water does not contain chlorine."** (The U.S. Council on Environmental Quality coordinates federal environmental efforts in developing environmental policies and initiatives.)

It may cause heart disease, too. Dr. Joseph Price wrote a highly controversial book in the late sixties entitled *Coronaries/Cholesterol/Chlorine*, and concluded *that nothing can negate the incontrovertible fact that the basic cause of arteriosclerosis, heart attacks, and stroke, is chlorine.*

So, why is chlorine so bad for us? Well, when chlorine is added to water, it combines with other natural compounds to form trihalomethanes (THMs), a chlorination byproduct. These chlorine byproducts trigger the production of free radicals in the body, which not only cause cell damage, but are highly carcinogenic.

But get this. You don't have to drink your chlorinated water to suffer from chlorine's ill effects. *Most of our exposure to chlorine—up to two-thirds, in fact—is due to inhalation of steam and skin absorption when showering.* The steam we inhale can contain up to 50 times the level of chemicals than tap water. How can this be? Well, chlorine and other contaminants vaporize much faster and at a lower temperature than water. Another thing you should know-- **inhaling chlorine is much more dangerous than *ingesting* it. Why? Because when we inhale chlorine gas it goes right to our bloodstream.**

And how about that other chemical that is added to our tap water in the name of good health? That's right, I'm talking about fluoride. That is the chemical that has been added to our municipal water systems in the name of preventing tooth decay.

But do you know what fluoride is? Fluoride is a by-product of both the aluminum and fertilizer industries. And instead of those industries having to dispose of this by-product—one which contains lead, cadmium, arsenic, and other toxins, by the way—they can dispose of it in our water systems in the name of good health!

However, some believe that fluoride is one of the most toxic substances on the planet earth. **Initially not tested as a carcinogen, tests later showed that fluoride caused both liver and bone cancer in laboratory animals.** In 1992, scientists found Alzheimer's-like symptoms in lab animals exposed to the chemical. **And in the same year an article in the *Journal of American Medicine* drew a correlation between drinking fluoridated water and an increase in hip fractures.**

What did the research show? In both 1995 and 2000 separate studies showed that putting fluoride in water did little to prevent tooth decay anyway. As a matter of fact in order to prevent tooth decay, fluoride has to be put directly on our teeth via a product like toothpaste.

So now that we think fluoride in our drinking water doesn't prevent tooth decay, do we know what it does do? Sure, but the news isn't good. During the 1990s alone, when the effects of fluoride on health drew a lot of attention and dollars, different studies suggested that fluoridated water causes learning disabilities, motor skill dysfunctions, and results in a lower IQ for children. Other studies showed a connection between fluoride and arthritis, Down's syndrome, chronic fatigue, fibromyalgia, and thyroid abnormalities.

Toxins in Our Water

Consider these facts when it comes to toxins we encounter in our water:

- Most wastewater treatment plants are not sophisticated enough to remove the synthetic chemicals found in drugs and toiletries before the water is recycled. This is why synthetic chemicals, pesticides, antibiotics, and drugs can be found in public water supplies.

- Did you know that your toothpaste, dishwashing liquid, and certain soaps contain a chemical called triclosan? So what's the problem? People who use these products with water that has been treated with chlorine are exposed to chloroform gas, the product of chlorine and triclosan meeting. The gas is absorbed through the skin or lungs, and is thought to cause cancer, depression, and problems with the liver.

- Tap water is often contaminated with Teflon, which is thought to cause birth defects and developmental problems in children.

- A rocket fuel called perchlorate can be found in the tap water of more than 20 million Americans. The same substance that is used in air bags, safety flares, and fireworks, this chemical has been found to cause thyroid dysfunction, cancer, and can harm the proper development of growing fetuses.

Antibiotics and Growth Hormones

Before you make dinner tonight, take a good look at your meat. It looks pretty innocent sitting there in its plastic-wrapped package, doesn't it? But it's what you *can't* see that's dangerous. Farmers routinely use both antibiotics and growth hormones in chicken, beef, pork, and other meats. And quite simply, these are not good for the consumer.

Let's talk a little bit about antibiotics first. The reasons for farmers using them are probably pretty evident. The use of antibiotics means that their stock stays less diseased without having to go to great lengths. **Using antibiotics allows farmers to raise more stock and keep it in closer quarters without it getting as sickly.**

It's interesting, really, that doctors are hesitant to prescribe antibiotics to their human patients unless they are really needed. Why? Because overuse of antibiotics causes drug-resistant bugs. And that's not good for anyone!

But while we are all being very conscious of the antibiotics we take first hand, we are a little more lax with our *second-hand consumption*. After all, the antibiotics that livestock consume do the same thing. They create drug-resistant bugs. And these are bugs that even our strongest medicine can't cure!

What about growth hormones? The reason for farmers using growth hormones should be extremely evident. It takes a lot less time to get livestock fattened up and ready for consumption. **Consider this: In**

1940, it took *four months* to grow a three-pound chicken. But in 1990, thanks (or no thanks, as you'll soon come to see) to estrogenic chemicals added to chicken feed, it took a *mere six weeks*. Great for the farmer, maybe, but not so great for us. How come?

When these cows and chickens laden with growth promoters are eaten by consumers, these chemicals interfere with our delicate hormone balance. This can cause a whole host of hormone issues, not to mention dreaded weight gain!

Antibiotics in Our Food Chain

- Americans consume about three million pounds of antibiotics every year.

- The animals chicken and cattle consume more than 24 million pounds.

- The problem? Dosing livestock with antibiotics can breed bacteria resistant to drugs.

- The antibiotics in our food supply destroy the good bacteria in our intestines, which weakens our immune system and allows more toxins to enter the body.

Prescription Medicines, Vaccines, and the Dentist

Okay, so now you have a good idea of the toxins that surround you in your environment, as well as those that are present in your food and water.

And I'm sure you are probably thinking that the medical community is one area that is, and should be, toxin free. The prescription drugs we take, the vaccines we receive, and the dental work we experience is all safe, right?

Wrong.

The fact is—and this is hard to believe considering that medicine is designed to protect our health—the drugs we take, the fillings we get at the dentist, and the vaccines we routinely give our children are full of toxins that overtax our bodies and cause poor health. Ironic, isn't it, considering that these very things are designed to protect us.

Prescription Drugs

Let's spend a little time talking about prescription drugs. It is a commonly held belief that people are living longer these days thanks to prescription drugs. Consider this: at the turn of the century the average lifespan was about 40 years. What is it today? Try 80!

That's quite a difference, but are drugs really the reason for our longevity? Or could it be our longevity has something to do with modern medical improvements and technology, improved food and beverage sanitation, less crowding, new and improved heating methods, and cleaner sewage systems? In general, our creature comforts have improved since the turn of the century, making it easier to live longer. So let's not be too quick to give prescription drugs all the credit. In fact, a former United States Public Health Service official named Anthony Cortese found that 90% of the reduction in the death rate occurred *before* the introduction of antibiotics and vaccines, mostly due to the above-mentioned reasons.

But when you look at the sheer volume of new prescription drugs out there, not to mention the way they are marketed and advertised, it's really hard to believe that they aren't the reason for our longer life spans. Just turn on your television or open a magazine and you'll be bombarded with ads for drugs that claim to cure everything from social shyness to the inability to pay attention. Indeed, there's a pill out there to cure every ill, some of which were probably not seen as diseases just a short time ago!

Would you believe that the pharmaceutical industry spends $2 billion per year making us believe that drugs are the answer to all our problems? But here's the truth. Prescription drugs are strong chemical agents with a host of side effects, toxicities, and interactions with other drugs. *Prescription drugs are dangerous.*

Consider this: In a medical report called "Death by Medicine" done in 2003, Drs. Gary Null, Carolyn Dean, Martin Feldman, Debora Rasio, and Dorothy Smith found that approximately 106,000 deaths occurred per year as a result of prescription drugs. We all want a quick fix to our problems, and it seems we feel the same way when it comes to our health. And sure, there's probably a pill out there that will fix your high cholesterol, heart problems, swollen joints, or bad mood. Unfortunately, these drugs also come with side effects and toxicities.

And here's something else to think about. Drugs don't *fix* your health problems. They just *cover up* the symptoms. In order to be truly healthy, you need to go to the root of the problem.

Don't get me wrong. I'm not saying there's never a place for drugs. What I'm saying is that they are over-used in general, and should only be used as a last resort. Is there a non-drug solution to your medical problem? There most likely is. But sadly, you won't likely find out from your medical doctor. Their medical school training most likely did not include non-drug approaches to most health issues. So what does this mean? Quite simply, it places the responsibility on each of us to seek out safer solutions to getting well and staying well.

Just as food crops grown in poor soil yield inferior food, vulnerable to pests and disease infestation, the same thing happens to our bodies. Can you imagine how badly your car would run if you put contaminated gasoline in it? If you are taking prescription drugs, you are asking your body to do a job it wasn't created to do.

The quickly increasing numbers of degenerative diseases in the USA tells us we had better rethink our approach to wellness *before it's too late*. Your body has built-in healing power. In many cases, you don't need toxic drugs to be well. You simply need to engage your innate healing power, which can make repairs to the damaged areas and keep you cleaner and running smoother. Symptoms begin to subside, normal function is restored, and often people are able to wean off the toxic medications they have taken for years. Yes, you *can* live a healthy life, in many cases prescription-free, and a little later we're going to tell you how.

In the meantime, let's talk about another issue in the medical world: vaccines.

Vaccines

No doubt, vaccines have proved handy during emergency medical epidemics when they've been used to get things under control.

But are vaccines always safe? The answer is no.

However, let's get into a little more detail here. It's not really the vaccine itself that isn't safe. It's the additives in the vaccine. Common vaccine additives include mercury, aluminum, formaldehyde, sulfites, and antifreeze. Not exactly materials your body is psyched to break down.

As a matter of fact, these additives have been linked to a large number of problems, including brain and nerve damage, autism, and ADHD. It's unfortunate that most people agree to have their children vaccinated without realizing that these toxic chemicals are used as preservatives and "adjuvants," which prolong the immune system response. I mean, how many parents do you know who would willingly inject their children with these toxins? The problem is that most parents *don't know* these toxins accompany the antigen in the vaccine.

Could the drug companies make their vaccines *without* additives like mercury? You bet. But that would mean making vaccines in single doses, which is a much more expensive proposition for drug companies. Much better for them that they should continue to argue about the uncertainty of the dangers of vaccine additives.

Your Teeth and Toxins

Okay, a trip to the dentist should be safe enough, right? Think again! From the fluoride treatments you receive in the dental chair, to the mercury fillings in your teeth, to the nickel used in your root canal, going to the dentist can be a very toxic experience!

As a matter of fact, you need a root canal like, well, you need a hole in your head! During root canals the heavy metal nickel is frequently used. And this heavy metal is no joke! Nickel is associated with health problems such as headaches, irritability, seizures, depression, heart arrhythmia, eczema, diarrhea, bladder irritation, arthritis, endometriosis, ulcers, low blood pressure, cirrhosis of the liver, neck ache, nasal polyps, chronic fatigue, insomnia, autoimmune disease, cancer, and anaphylactic shock and death.

The other heavy metal often used at your dentist is mercury. Mercury has been in the news a lot lately as it pertains to the level in seafood. But did you know that the amount of mercury that you receive in one filling greatly outweighs the amount the FDA tells you to avoid in seafood?

While many of today's dentists still use mercury, with all the bad press and controversy mercury has generated, it's not difficult to find a dentist who uses other alternatives. How do you tell a mercury filling from a non-mercury filling? Mercury fillings are silver-to-black. As I've mentioned before, mercury is a heavy metal and powerful toxin that causes issues like mood swings, inability to concentrate, headaches, light sensitivity, loss of smell and taste, tremors, asthma, ulcers, bloating and gas, frequent night urination, constipation, rashes, arthritis, poor circulation, muscle cramps, fatigue, allergies, hypoglycemia, multiple sclerosis, and fibromyalgia.

Fluoride

When you go to the dentist to have your teeth cleaned, your teeth will most likely be brushed with fluoridated toothpaste. You may even receive a fluoride treatment, in which your teeth are coated with the chemical to prevent them from decaying.

But what's the payoff? First of all, let's consider what fluoride is. It's a byproduct of the aluminum and fertilizer industries. In its gas form, it is used not only to make bombs, but as a pesticide. Is it worth it to put it on your teeth? Or in your body?

Fluoride is suspected to cause motor skill dysfunctions, learning disabilities, arthritis, Down's syndrome, and certain cancers. It has also been demonstrated to inhibit the uptake of iodine by the thyroid, thereby causing hypothyroidism. Actually in the 1950s it was used as a prescription for hyperthyroid because of its anti-thyroid affects. While fluoride applied directly to the teeth has been shown to prevent decay, I would say that the things that go along with it just aren't worth it, wouldn't you?

CHAPTER 5

HOW TOXINS ARE DESTROYING YOUR HEALTH

What 98% of Doctors Don't Know

A Deeper Look into Chronic Illness

> *"When Kayla (age 6) came to Nutrition Wellness Center she'd been diagnosed with Lyme disease and lymphoma. After one month on the detox program her energy level has improved quite a bit; but it's not a hyper energy like bouncing off the walls; it's a good energy like children should have. Before, she could only walk a block or two before she'd complain about her feet and legs being sore and tired. Now she can walk about two miles without complaining about her feet being sore. Emotionally, she has leveled out and is more cheerful.*
>
> *"The specialist (ear, nose, and throat doctor) recently examined her after six weeks of nutritional and detox therapy, and he said there is no lump (lymphoma); her neck is completely normal. We are all so happy!*
> —Kayla
> Dunedin, Florida
> (Reported by her Grandmother)

Most of us in environmental and alternative medicine know the DIRECT effects toxins have on specific organs and tissues. For example: pesticides in the brain interfere with brain chemistry and can cause inflammation and tissue damage. This means pesticides can interfere with serotonin and dopamine levels. That's why several studies have associated pesticides with Parkinson's disease. Fluoride in the thyroid, according to many published studies interferes with thyroid metabolism, thyroid function and contributes to hypothyroidism. The list goes on, but I think you get the idea. Toxins in tissues can cause biochemical malfunctions, inflammation and even tissue damage.

The missing piece of this 'toxin = dis-ease' puzzle is what I will expound upon next. Pay very close attention to what you are about to read. Many, if not most of the conventional and alternative practitioners are NOT aware of this MAJOR piece of the puzzle!

The information in this chapter may well be the missing pieces of the puzzle for many chronically ill people.

Our immune system is the valiant defender against the daily assaults by toxins, when it is working right. It is a complex system made up of many different components that work together and defines our degree of health or illness. The ability of the immune system to detoxify toxins plays a critical role in maintaining our health. Failure or lack of this ability to detoxify toxins results in health issues such as obesity, chronic fatigue syndrome, fibromyalgia, brain fog, depression, anxiety, poor circulation, leaky gut syndrome, irritable bowel syndrome, attention deficit disorder, hyperactivity, autism, and autoimmune disorders such as rheumatoid arthritis, eczema, diabetes type II, and multiple sclerosis.

There are hundreds if not thousands of toxins that we are exposed to everyday. Generally, they fall into two main categories: 1) biological toxins and 2) man-made toxins. Biological toxins or biotoxins for short are toxic substances that are produced by living organisms. On the other hand, man-made toxins are just that- any substance made by man that has a poisonous or harmful effect on us.

Genetics Role in Our Body Ecology

Biological toxins are produced by a variety of organisms found in the air, on land and in water environments. What makes biotoxins so toxic is their water like structure. It allows them to more easily travel across cell membranes and go from cell to cell. They do not need blood to travel. It's their ability to jump from cell to cell that makes them so dangerous. Certain toxins move throughout the body very rapidly going directly from cell to cell. So, a toxin that may have been inhaled into the lungs can end up in our heart, gut, liver, gallbladder, skin, glands and even our muscles and brain tissue as well.

Microorganisms such as bacteria, fungus, mold, yeast and algae comprise a large portion of this group. You may already be familiar with some of these, for example, the bacteria group streptococcus (strep throat). Standard medical treatment is to prescribe a course of antibiotics. The problem is the drug may kill the organism but it will not get rid of the toxin produced by it. That job is left up to the body's immune system. Clearing the toxin eliminates the lingering symptoms in healthy people. Your body can do this because you have genes that are responsible for instructing the body to recognize and tag toxins which are then eliminated usually through the liver. If toxins aren't tagged as foreign invaders, the liver WILL NOT detoxify the toxins. This can happen if the genes responsible for detoxifying are turned off (like a lamp or a light switch). Turning genes on or off, i.e., gene switching is primarily caused by toxins. The consequences are similar as for those with actual genetic defects. The difference is, with gene switching, the process can be turned around given the proper corrective actions and enough time.

Worst Case Scenario

Failure to clear these toxins, whether biotoxins or man made, can also come from bad genetics. This genetic defect (designated HLA DR genotype) renders the body incapable of recognizing a toxin as something foreign to the body. It will not be metabolized or excreted and people stay ill long after their exposure to the toxin has stopped. About 25% of the American population has this genetic defect. They are affected the most and usually develop long standing chronic health issues. Sadly, they are often sent on a merry-go-round of health care practitioners and are put on multiple medications which are used to band-aid the symptoms without treating the cause. Welcome to "sick care" in America. Ultimately, this downward spiral of chronic ill health dooms them to be sick for the rest of their lives. This does not necessarily have to be your fate. If you are diligent, you can find someone who understands this process and is knowledgeable in proper detoxification methods. Preventive maintenance is the critical key to staying healthy. It is a life long commitment.

Too Much of a Bad Thing

At the other end of the spectrum is the segment of the American population that has the genetic capability to detoxify and eliminate toxins. The good news is that it is the case for the majority of the population. Regrettably, that genetic capability does not always translate into maintainable good health. The primary reason is toxic overload. To truly understand this we need to look back to the era of the Industrial Revolution. Less than 100 years ago, generation after generation had only a small segment of toxins they were being exposed to on a regular basis. Our detoxification system could handle that in most instances. Along came the Industrial Revolution and with it more than 70,000 new man made chemicals were introduced into our daily lives. "Better living through chemistry" defined the modern age. Speed and convenience became the measurement by which our standard of living was graded. From transportation to healthcare, every area of our daily lives was touched in some way by these new chemicals. Little did the public realize the true cost or the magnitude of these toxic stresses.

Today, our body's detoxification system is so overloaded from decades of exposure that breakdown and failure of this system is occurring daily in people across the United States. This is being reflected in the emergence of new chronic illnesses like chronic fatigue syndrome, fibromyalgia, autism and ADD in adults and children alike. Toxic overload does not happen overnight. It is continuous exposure on a daily basis for years at a time that overloads and overwhelms the body's detoxification pathways. In other words, more is coming in than is going out resulting in the system breaking down. Fortunately, in many cases, persons with toxic overload have the greatest and quickest recovery time when the toxic overload is properly addressed. Frequently, even in a few weeks to a couple of months, a detoxification program will produce results in reducing symptoms, depending on the toxic overload.

In summary, we are products of our heredity (genetics) and our environment. Our world is vastly different from that of our ancestors. We eat, breathe and live in our modern environment, making ingestion of toxins a part of everyday life. Our genetic makeup and the environment determine three main reasons why people cannot detoxify toxins; 1) gene switching, 2) genetic defect and 3) toxin overload. Which one are you?

Where the Dominos Start to Fall

To understand what happens in our body when it is exposed to a toxin, we begin with the fat cell. Fat cells are more than padding on our waistlines and hips. They are dynamic, hard working cells that produce hormones and chemicals that influence our immune system. As most of us already know, many toxins are stored in fat tissue. A recent study, done by the EPA, analyzed 25,000 fat biopsies which revealed toxic chemicals in 100% of the samples tested. The list of chemicals found included styrene, dichlorobenzene, xylene, ethyl phenol and benzene. These are known cancer causing agents! What happens in a fat cell is, often, these highly mobile toxins will attach themselves to the outside part of a fat cell call the "receptor" (landing site) on the cell membrane. The receptor is an area or landing site that is located on the cell surface that normally binds with a specific molecule, hormone or antibody. In the case of a toxin landing there, it will turn on genes in the fat cells to make "inflammation" chemicals that circulate throughout the body. How does it do this? Toxins can transmit a signal from the outside of the cell membrane to the nucleus of the cell. This allows the toxins to activate the genes inside the cell. Thus, genetic warfare begins.

The Good, the Bad and the Uncontrolled

Fat cells can make cytokines. Cytokines are proteins that communicate with other cells to turn on and help control the immune responses, i.e., inflammation chemicals. An increase in cytokines causes an increase in inflammation. This can happen anywhere in the body. For example, increased cytokine levels on our capillaries attract white blood cells. This leads to reduced or restricted blood flow to the area and lower oxygen levels as well. A person can experience symptoms such as muscle cramps, fatigue and shortness of breath.

Increased cytokines can cause other symptoms which includes headaches, muscle aches, hard time concentrating and even your temperature can vary.

Your immune system is like the military organization with all the branches. The National Guard, Army, Navy, Air Force and

Marines are ready to do battle against foreign invaders. The immune system has different organizational units, like each military branch, that performs specific roles in defense of our country, in this case, our body. Sometimes they can perform their job too well and problems occur. Therefore, a continuous out of control production of cytokines is like pouring gasoline on the fire or pushing down on the gas pedal in your car and not letting up. Something will eventually blow. The system wasn't designed for an out of control continuous production of inflammation chemicals eventually spreading throughout the body.

Sick All Over

As with any military operation, communication networks are critical to the success of any mission. Enter the courier known as MMP-9(matrix metalloproteinase-9).Increased cytokine levels and inflammation chemicals affect immune response associated chemicals such as MMP-9. MMP-9 acts like a courier delivering inflammatory elements from your blood to the brain, lungs, muscles, nerves and joints. So, if things weren't bad enough with the out of control inflammation, now a chemical that acts as an accelerated delivery system to other tissues or parts of the body comes into play and speeds up the whole inflammatory process.

Fatigue, Muscle Cramps and Joint Pain

Infrastructure and support services such as power, water, food, and medical supplies are vital for smooth operations. Creating and maintaining supply routes (roads) are equally critical. The body makes a substance called vascular endothelial growth factor (VEGF). In healthy people, VEGF stimulates blood vessel growth and dilates blood vessels thus bringing in more oxygen to capillaries and tissues.

This is like creating roads and widening them (road improvements) as needed to deliver goods and services. High cytokine levels decrease the production of VEGF which in turn affects normal blood flow. Low VEGF means reduced blood flow to our organs and capillaries causing less oxygen and vital nutrients to be delivered to them. This situation is similar to corrosion in pipes not allowing the proper water flow through the faucet. People with decreased VEGF can not deliver the proper amount of oxygen needed to meet any increased demand such as with exercise or more than usual activity. Ever hear the caution "check with your doctor before starting any exercise program"? When our oxygen level is decreased what follows are symptoms like fatigue, brain fog, joint pain, muscle cramps and shortness of breath.

Autoimmune Problems

High cytokine levels are particularly problematic for people who are dealing with biotoxin induced illness and autoimmune issues. Your immune response systems are already on full alert and mobilizing the military troops to engage the enemy. In the heat of battle (increased inflammation), the command post is infiltrated and orders are sent out to turn on autoimmune genes. The troops go berserk and attack their own units or their allies. In other words, our own antibodies attack our organs. This can show up as digestive problems, circulation issues including fertility problems or neurological diseases just to name a few. How does this happen?

Leaky Gut and Irritable Bowel Syndrome

Biotoxicity and increased cytokines can cause increases in antigliadin antibodies (AGA).Gliadin is a protein contained in gluten. Gluten is a protein found in wheat, barley, oats and rye. Gliadin is not normally absorbed in the body in healthy people. If your small intestines happen to absorb the gliadin molecule it will treat it as a foreign invader and attack it by setting off the cytokine alarm. Antigliadin antibodies (AGA) are made and released. Increased AGA is associated with leaky gut syndrome, irritable bowel syndrome and major digestive problems. Avoiding gluten containing foods is highly recommended in these cases.

Circulation Problems and Infertility

Another antibody called anticardiolipin antibody (ACLA) may show up in people with biotoxin illness. It is not normally found in healthy people either. Reduced circulation in small blood vessels, unusual clotting problems and fertility problems (1st trimester miscarriages) can be associated with ACLA levels.

Multiple Sclerosis and Nerve Problems

Biotoxin illness and high cytokines can increase myelin basic protein (MBP) antibodies. Myelin is the insulation around your nerve fibers and is important for rapid nerve pulse transmission. Increased MBP antibodies are associated with multiple sclerosis (MS) and nerve problems.

Weight Gain and Diabetes

Unfortunately, high cytokine levels and the accompanying inflammation don't stop there. Obesity and Type II diabetes are affecting more and more Americans in younger and younger age groups. So what's the connection? The culprits are damaged receptor sites (or landing areas) in the brain and cells all over the body. Receptor sites are like landing pads on the outside of the cell membrane where hormones, for example, land on a cell to complete a communication or cause an action to occur in that cell. Think of a hormone molecule as a plug on an electrical cord and the receptor site as an electrical outlet. Damaged receptor sites means communication is blocked and there is failure of the receptors to function normally. No juice-no action. This, in turn will lead to various types of hormone resistances including leptin and insulin.

Let's look at the hormone leptin, for instance. Leptin is a hormone produced by fat cells. Its purpose is to communicate to the brain (hypothalamus area) to turn off "hunger". For this communication to occur, leptin goes to leptin receptor sites in the hypothalamus. If these receptor sites are damaged, no communication takes place. It is as if leptin is calling the brain but the brain is not answering, no matter how loudly leptin is shouting. The result is leptin resistance. Leptin resistance is failure of the leptin receptors to function normally. Too much leptin in the bloodstream increases storage of fatty acids in fat cells causing fat weight gain. Similarly, when insulin receptors are damaged, too much insulin remains in the blood and leads to insulin resistance. Insulin is not being utilized by the cells thus contributing to the development of Type II diabetes and weight gain. The heartbreak of hormone resistance results in the body's inability to control weight by normal means like diet and exercise. In other words, that triple cheeseburger will stick to your ribs, waistline and any other parts of your body.

A Key Hormone Having a Major Effect on Our Health

Your body is like a huge corporation. It is very complex and it has developed systems to run the company smoothly and efficiently. The brain acts as corporate headquarters dictating policies and procedures, directing operations and acts as a central clearinghouse for processing vast amounts of information. This command center is called the hypothalamus. It ultimately regulates the whole neuroendocrine (nerve-hormone) system. When cytokine levels become too high, damage to leptin receptor sites in the hypothalamus can occur. This, in turn, can cause a lowered production of an important hormone called MSH (melanocyte stimulating hormone).

MSH is produced in the brain and regulates over twenty different functions. Low MSH levels can cause a number of systems to literally go haywire, affecting our immune system, gut, sex drive and sleep, just to name a few.

You Are Just Getting Old ---- Or Are You?

When MSH production is reduced your pituitary gland function diminishes. The pituitary gland produces several major hormones all of which are influenced by MSH. Low MSH levels cause the pituitary gland to produce less anti-diuretic hormone (ADH). Low ADH may make you feel thirsty, have frequent urination and even lead you to be more susceptible to shock from static electricity. Reduction of MSH can make the pituitary lower its production of sex hormones, hence, lower sex drive. Changes in ACTH (adrenocorticotropic hormone) and cortisol levels will also occur. ACTH is produced by the pituitary gland. Low ACTH levels stimulate the cortex (outside portion) of the adrenal gland to produce cortisol. During the onset of illness, the pituitary can cause higher levels of ACTH and cortisol initially, but then these levels will drop to excessively low levels later on. How does this affect the body? High levels of ACTH or cortisol

levels may show up as thinning skin, easy bruising, weight gain especially on the face, upper back and trunk, high blood pressure, thirst and frequent urination. Subsequently, when these hormone levels fall a person may experience weakness, fatigue, loss of appetite, weight loss, nausea/vomiting, abdominal pain, dizziness, low blood pressure, skin color changes and electrolyte imbalances.

Chronic Sinus Problems and Slow Healing

MSH plays a critical role in the health and functions of the mucous tissues in the sinuses and gut. It also plays a major role in healthy skin function. Low MSH levels can cause groups of antibiotic resistant Staphylococcus bacteria to build up in your sinus membranes. This is not good news. These bacteria make substances that worsen both high cytokine levels and low MSH levels. This can lead to prolonged illness from infections because white blood cell response time is affected and healing time is dramatically slowed down.

Leaky Gut and Chronic Pain

Endorphins are 'pleasure chemicals,' and their effects are well-known to runners who experience a 'natural high' after running. Pain experienced in healthy people as a 'level 4,' (on a 1-10 scale) would be sensed as a 'level 8,' by someone with low endorphin levels. These are the individuals who suffer from fibromyalgia, muscle aches and pains, and general all over discomfort.

Insomnia

How many adults over age 40 have difficulty falling asleep or staying asleep? When MSH levels are low, our pineal gland cannot make a hormone called melatonin, which is crucial for normal sleep patterns. In addition to regulating biological rhythms, melatonin is considered a powerful anti-oxidant. Reduced melatonin levels also speed up aging. Once MSH levels are restored, melatonin production resumes and restful sleep is once again a part of life. Without regular restful sleep, all healing processes are hindered. Prescription and over-the-counter sleep drugs are not the answer and often compound the problem with the addition of more toxins the body must defend against.

Final Thoughts

Our bodies are marvelous feats of engineering and organization with the capacity to heal itself given the right conditions. We live in the information age and have the tools to gain the knowledge needed to take charge of our health. Many of the terms used in this chapter may be new to you and can be a tongue twister. But, there is not one reason I can think of that would prevent you from learning if you truly wanted to. It is my deepest hope that you take the information in this book and use it to help change your health and change your life. This chapter should shed some light on why a detox is NOT just a colon cleanse. I would hope this book gives you a better understanding of the whole picture in body symptoms and tissues affected by toxins. A colon cleanse may give you some temporary relief but it doesn't handle the above issues discussed. Therefore it becomes a temporary band-aid and nothing more.

Search for the underlying causes not just band-aid the symptoms. Become partners with a health care provider that works with you and is not afraid to explore different approaches. New research is being published everyday and can open up new possibilities for health care revolutions. Begin the path to becoming the healthiest you can be by asking the question, "HOW TOXIC ARE YOU?"

CHAPTER 6

DETOXIFY YOUR LIFE

Product Dangers and Smarter Shopping Choices

"Over the past few years I have had problems with joint pain and swelling, an intermittent tremor of my right hand, low energy level, fatigue, and insomnia. After being convinced to try this approach to wellness, following the appropriate diet and supplement regime, I have eradicated all of these problems. My color has improved; people ask me what I've done and say I look so much better! I even lost 10 pounds, not a goal, but very much appreciated. Thank you so much!"

—Jan, R.N.

Burr Oak, Michigan

When you consider that toxins are all around us, the situation at hand can seem pretty bleak. After all, toxins are on our table, in our water, and in our clothing, furniture, medicines, and even in the fillings in our teeth. They are *every*where!

So how do you avoid the synthetic chemicals that surround us? Well, I admit that, unless you live in a cave, it is impossible to avoid all of them. However, with certain smart lifestyle choices, it is possible to cut down on the amount of toxins you expose yourself to. Ridding yourself of toxins requires a two-pronged approach. The first thing you must do is take steps to ensure that you come into contact with fewer toxins in the future. This means paying attention to the food you eat, the water you drink, the personal care products you use, and the cleaning products you have around the house. The second, and equally important, step is to rid yourself of the toxins that your body is *already* carrying and has accumulated over years. Detoxification is where I come in, and I'm going to devote a whole chapter to that later. In the meantime, let's talk about some ways that you can diminish your contact with toxins on a day-to-day basis.

Your Healthy Home

We've already discussed in detail whether we should be concerned with household toxins. The answer is a resounding yes! By now you know that the biggest culprit of toxin exposure is in your own home. Toxic household products are being produced for our daily living which has significant impact on our health and environment. These products are made from materials and substances that can cause cancer, birth defects, change in genetic structure, and can deplete our immune system.

What's the best way to protect yourself against toxic products? Why, read the labels, of course! Be sure to look for signal words placed by the federal government to protect and inform you of the potential impact on your environment. Annie Berthold-Bond's book, *Better Basics for the Home*, explains these signal words to watch out for.

"POISON/DANGER means something very toxic; only a few drops could kill you. WARNING means moderately toxic; as little as a teaspoonful can kill. CAUTION denotes a product that is less toxic; two tablespoons to a cup could kill you."

I encourage you to experiment and eventually make the change to practical, hands on, day-to-day, non-toxic, environmentally safe home cleaning products. This sidebar on healthy home product solutions is a great place to start!

Healthy Home Products Solutions

The following are samples of basic, safe cleaning solutions:

KITCHEN CLEANER
Place 1 t Borax, 1/2 t washing soda, 2 T vinegar, and 1/4 to 1/2 t vegetable oil-based liquid soap in a spray bottle. Add 2 cups very hot tap water and shake gently until the minerals have dissolved. Spray onto the surface you are cleaning and wipe off.

GREASE CUTTING SPRAY CLEANER
Use 1/2 t washing soda, 2 T vinegar, 1/4 t vegetable oil-based liquid soap, (such as Seventh Generation brand) and 2 cups of very hot water. Mix and apply.

SCOURING POWDER
Plain baking soda, applied with a damp sponge, works beautifully. It can leave a residue, however, if not rinsed thoroughly.

HAND DISHWASHING LIQUID
Use vegetable oil-based soap just as you would a commercial brand. When you first open the bottle, add a couple of drops of liquid Vitamin E or cut open a Vitamin E capsule and pour in the contents. This helps protect against nitrosamine (a carcinogen) from chemicals in the soap.

OVEN CLEANER

Generously sprinkle the bottom of the oven with water, cover grime with baking soda, and sprinkle on more water. Let it sit overnight and wipe up in the morning with a mild abrasive pad. With a bit of vegetable oil-based soap on a sponge, wash the sides and top of the oven and inside the door, as well as any remaining grease or baking soda on the bottom. Rinse thoroughly. For tougher jobs, use a small box of baking soda and 1/4 cup washing soda, applying the washing soda particularly to burned-on grease. Extra rinsing will be required.

WINDOWS

Put 1/4 to 1/2 t vegetable oil-based liquid soap, 3 T vinegar, and 2 cups water in a spray bottle and shake it up. Use just like a commercial window cleaner. If windows are very greasy, use 1/4 t vegetable oil-based liquid soap, 3 T vinegar, 1/4 t washing soda, and 2 cups very hot water to dissolve the minerals.

FLOORS

Put 1/8 cup vegetable oil-based liquid soap and 1/2 cup vinegar in a bucket and fill with warm water, swirling to mix. Or add 1 cup vinegar to a pail of water.

WALLS

Mix 1/8 to 1/4 cup vegetable oil-based liquid soap and 2 gallons of water in a bucket until sudsy. Wash the walls with a sponge. For wallpaper, rub off smudges with a slice or two of white bread.

DUSTING

Make your furniture polish cloth for wood furniture by mixing 1/2 t olive oil and 1/4 cup vinegar or lemon juice in a bowl. Dip a soft cotton rag into the mixture and dust and polish your furniture with it. You can reuse the cloth many times.

BATHROOM

Mix 1/4 cup baking soda with enough vegetable oil-based liquid soap to make a paste. Apply with a damp sponge, scrub, and rinse thoroughly.

TOILET BOWL CLEANER
Pour 1 cup of Borax into the toilet and leave it overnight. In the morning flush it without scrubbing. If you don't want to leave it overnight, use 1 cup of borax and 1/4 cup of vinegar, let it rest a few hours, scrub, and brush. Or substitute 1/2 cup baking soda and clean immediately.

TOILET BOWL DISINFECTANT
Mix a few drops of Australian tea tree oil and 2 cups of water in a spray bottle. Spray into the toilet bowl. Leave it for a few minutes, then scrub.

TO KEEP DRAINS CLEAR
Pour 1/4 cup washing soda down the drain each week and rinse with hot water, or just pour 1/4 cup of vinegar down the drain. For a little more action, pour 1/2 cup of baking soda and 3 cups boiling water or 1/2 cup of baking soda and 1/2 cup vinegar and let the mixture gurgle for 15 minutes. Then rinse with hot water.

LAUNDRY
Several commercial laundry detergents are available such as Ecover and Life Tree. For extra-dirty loads, add 1/2 cup or more of washing soda. To prevent static cling, add 1/4 cup of vinegar to the rinse cycle.

LAUNDRY BOOSTERS
To a full load add any one of the following:

    1/2 cup baking soda
    1/4 cup vinegar
    1 T odor-fresh zeolite*
    1/4 cup Borax
    1/2 cup washing soda—this can also be used as a bleach alternative

*(zeolite is a natural mineral collected from where volcanic rocks and ash layers react with alkaline groundwater. Also used commercially in water purification and production of medical-grade oxygen, because of its ability to trap impurities, also now available as a nutritional supplement to bind toxins in the gut)

Sitting Pretty—the Healthy Way

Not only are we exposing ourselves to toxic chemicals in the everyday cleaning and maintenance of our homes, we are also slathering them on our skin and bodies every time we put on suntan lotion, face and body creams, makeup, and other personal care products. Would you believe that personal care products can contain chemicals like pesticides, preservatives, plastics, fluoride, and artificial scents? To be sure, all of these things are designed to make the product look and smell better, and last longer. The downside? You are being exposed to unhealthy chemicals you could certainly do without! How's this for a statistic? *The National Institute of Occupational Safety and Health has found more than 2,500 toxic chemicals in cosmetics.* Even worse, these chemicals have been proven to cause eye and skin irritation, tumors, as well as reproductive and biological issues.

And here's yet another statistic. During the course of the day most of us are exposed to more than 200 different chemicals all in the name of personal hygiene and beauty. You read it right—200 chemicals!

But by paying attention to the products you use on your body, you can dramatically slash the amount of chemicals you are being exposed to. That's good news!

But how do you know what chemicals are safe and which aren't? A good resource is a website maintained by the Environmental Working Group called Skin Deep (www.cosmeticsdatabase.com).

All you need to do is type in the name of the products you use, and it will tell you if any of the ingredients in that product are potential health threats.

Do You Know What's In Your Beauty Products?

Cosmetic: Talcum Powder
      Chemical: crystalline silica
      Health risk: known human carcinogen

Cosmetic: Shampoos that control itching and eczema
      Chemical: coal tar
      Health risk: Known human carcinogen

Cosmetic: Shampoos, nail treatments, moisturizing body bars
      Chemical: benzyl violet 2
      Health risk: Carcinogen

Cosmetic: Menopause creams, hair-thinning serum, anti-dandruff shampoos, sun screens
      Chemical: formaldehyde
      Health risk: Probable carcinogen linked to breast cancer and abnormal growth of reproductive tissue

Cosmetic: Hair dye
      Chemical: lead acetate
      Health risk: Known carcinogen that can cause brain damage

Cosmetic: Dandruff shampoo
      Chemical: selenium sulfide
      Health risk: Carcinogen

Cosmetic: Skin moisturizers, nail polish
      Chemical: Phthalates
      Health risk: causes birth defects in male children

Cosmetic: Blush, mascara, lipstick, hair dye, powder, foundation, concealer, moisturizers, sun screens
    Chemical: parabens
    Heath risk: can cause breast cancer and birth abnormalities

Cosmetic: shampoo, body wash, bubble bath, and toothpaste
    Chemical: sodium lauryl sulfate
    Health risk: contains carcinogenic contaminants, increases the absorption of toxic chemicals

Cosmetic: Hairspray
    Chemical: butylene glycol
    Health risk: skin irritant

Cosmetic: Nail polish
    Chemical: zirconium
    Health risk: causes respiratory problems

Cosmetic: Toothpaste
    Chemical: potassium bromate
    Health risk: causes bleeding and inflammation of gums

Cosmetic: hair dye, astringent
    Chemical: nickel sulfate
    Health risk: skin irritant

Cosmetic: Dandruff shampoo
    Chemical: resorcinol
    Health risk: skin irritant

What's your best course of action? Choose your products carefully, ensuring that they are made by companies that sell natural, organic products. Is it going to take a little more time and money to make the right choices? You bet! But the health benefits you'll enjoy will be well worth it.

Here's a list of products I find safe:

Shampoo: Dessert Essence with lavender and tea tree oil, Aubrey shampoos and conditioners.

Toothpaste: Peelu Toothpaste, Tom's of Maine (without fluoride) toothpaste, hydrogen peroxide with 50% water, Baking soda (never use toothpaste with fluoride, or those stored in tin containers).

Deodorant: Nature's Gate brand, natural deodorant crystal stick, pure mineral salts with potassium sulfate and no aluminum, Aubrey pump or roll on, Tea Tree Oil by Jason Cosmetics, Apricot & E by Jason Cosmetics, Alvera Aloe & Almond Roll On, Alvera Aloe Herbal Roll On, Herbal Magic Unscented Roll On, Tom's of Maine Natural Anti-Perspirant Unscented, Tea Tree Deodorant by Thursday Plantation, Tea Tree Sport Deodorant by Thursday Plantation.

Mouthwash: Tom's Spearmint or Cinnamint Natural Mouthwash, Natural Dentist Herbal Mouth and Gum Therapy in mint or children flavors, Thursday Plantation Tea Tree/Cinnamon, hydrogen peroxide 1/2 strength.

Suntan Lotions: Nature's Gate Suntan Lotion SPF 8, Nature's Gate Sun Block SPF 15.

Shaving: Electric razor, straight razor with castile liquid soap by Desert Essence, Burt's Bees' Shaving Soap in Rum Spice.

Soap: Dr. Bronner's Castile Liquid Soap, Kiss My Face Olive Oil Bar, Chandrika Ayurvedic Soap.

Hand/Body Lotion: Extra virgin olive oil, Burt's Bees' Buttermilk Lotion, Aubrey lotions.

Fragrances: 100% pure essential oils that are free of isopropyl alcohol or IPA.

Cosmetics: Burt's Bees' or Kiss My Face brands.

Hair Dye: Herbatint Herbal Hair Color Gel

Lips: Desert Lip Rescue with Tea Tree Oil, Burt's Bees'.

Maintaining Healthy Teeth and Gums in a Toxic World

After reading this far you already know that something as innocent as brushing your teeth and visiting the dentist can be hazardous to your health! If you follow the normal regiment of dental care suggested by many dentists, you are exposing yourself to toxins such as mercury and fluoride. *Neither one of which belongs in your body!*

First let's talk about the daily care of your teeth and gums. Choose all-natural, fluoride-free toothpaste such as Tom's of Maine, which you can find in the health food section of most grocery stores. Brush your teeth after every meal as you normally would.

Now I'm going to introduce you to Neem Oil. What is Neem Oil? It is oil originally from the Neem tree in India that fights bacteria. So how do you use it? After you brush, put one or two drops of Neem Oil on a wet toothbrush and brush your teeth, gums, and tongue. Be sure not to rinse, although you can drink water as needed. Remember, most bacterial overgrowth starts in the mouth!

How about your trip to the dentist? Before you head over to the office, be sure to brush your teeth as usual and use your Neem Oil. This will help kill any bacteria on your teeth before your dentist or hygienist cleans the hardened bacteria, otherwise known as plaque, off your teeth. What happens if you don't brush with Neem Oil first? Well, when the dentist cleans your teeth you'll run the risk of swallowing the bacteria he's been knocking off your teeth. These bacteria will head toward and infect the vital organs in your body. Yuck!

After your dental appointment, I also recommend that you do the same procedure as above with your Neem Oil, as added protection twice a day for one week. Then resume to once per day. (if you cannot find Neem Oil, pure and made without solvents, call Nutrition Wellness Center (800) 222-3610 to order)

So how about all the other work done on your teeth at the dentist? Just say no to fluoride treatments, and be sure to use a dentist that uses material other than mercury and nickel in fillings and root canals. Remember, heavy metals belong in cars, not in your mouth! Heavy metals suppress the immune system and make it difficult for your body to naturally fight off infection from bacteria.

Get the Toxins off Your Table . . . and Out of Your Drinking Glass

We live in a toxic world where our food and water is laced with additives, dyes, pesticides, metals, and other chemicals. So what is the best way to get toxins off our tables and out of our bodies? *Prevention.*

Let's talk about the toxins in our food, first. Here are a few things we know. We know that 4 billion pounds of pesticides are used per year here in the United States. And we also know that recent studies have shown 50-70 chemical residues in the fatty tissues of ordinary Americans. Considering that our brains are 60% fat, this isn't the best of news!

In addition to pesticides, cattle and poultry farmers are adding to the problem by using synthetic fattening chemicals and heavy metals such as arsenic to increase their livestock's weight. Not only are these chemicals not good for us, they also make us fat by tampering with our hormonal systems.

So how do we fight the toxins on our table?

- **Avoid packaged foods, such as canned and processed foods. It may take a little more time and money, but it is well worth it to prepare as many meals from scratch as possible.**

- **Buy organic fruits, veggies, and meat, or grow or raise your own.**

- **If you buy meat, try to buy locally. And make sure that the meat is organic and free of antibiotics and growth hormones.**

Now that you have them off your table, take a look in your drinking glass. Chances are, if you drink municipal water, you are being exposed to dangerous chemicals such as fluoride, perchlorate, chlorine, and arsenic. And if you have well water you might not be that much better off. Pesticides might be your problem.

Water is the stuff of life. How to ensure that the water you and your family are drinking is doing you more good than harm?

- Find out if arsenic or other harmful contaminants are in your water supply. If they are, get the proper water purification system to treat your specific problem.

- Stop using pesticides on your lawn and garden, as they can leach into your water system.

- If you have chlorine in your water, take the first step of installing a point-of-entry filtration system, or an ozone or ultraviolet water filtration system, or a whole-house reverse osmosis system, to cut down on the amount of chlorine in your water.

- Buy organic bottled water, or spring water, preferably in non-plastic containers.

CHAPTER 7

THE MISSING LINK FOR WEIGHT LOSS

You CAN Become Thinner!
Making Weight Management EASIER!

> *"I was overweight for approximately 10 years. It put constraints on my activities and on my energy. Before meeting Dr. Martin, I'd followed a million different diets, and the weight would come and go, but no consistent weight loss. I first heard about Dr. Martin from my wife, after she'd done some research.*
>
> *"Since coming to Nutrition Wellness Center, I've lost 28 pounds, I've cleared toxins, and I feel a lot better. My energy has increased dramatically. My blood pressure is better. I feel better than I have in years!*
>
> *"A lot of people have noticed the changes—my business associates, friends, acquaintances, my wife, even my father, who's my staunchest critic, has noticed.*
>
> *"Nutrition Wellness Center is a great thing, all natural, no drugs involved, going about it the right way, doing it naturally. I will absolutely recommend Nutrition Wellness Center to others."*
>
> —Mitch
> Palm Harbor, Florida

> *"For 13 years no one could tell me why I was overweight, even though I exercised and ate the right diet. I would not lose one pound—we walked three miles per day.*
>
> *"I went to a lot of doctors, smart doctors, one spoke eight different languages, and none of them helped me lose weight. I went for 13 years to other doctors but they couldn't help me.*
>
> *"I know I was so overloaded with toxins, chemicals, and heavy metals. I spent between $80,000 to $100,000 on those other doctors. Dr. Martin told me once I started detoxing it would help my thyroid and liver, and they would function better (I did lose 20 pounds without exercising). Thank God we were able to find Dr. Martin."*
>
> —Debbie
> Plant City, Florida

Are toxins making you fat?

The United States has one of the most overweight populations in the world. Why? Could that have anything to do with the fact that we also produce the largest amount of synthetic chemicals?

I think so.

Low-calorie diets work for some people. But the vast majority of overweight Americans have other factors standing firm between them and their ideal weight. And guess what? These factors are *overlooked* by most weight-loss clinics, popular diets, and by most medical professionals.

When it comes to obesity, we've all heard the phrase, "It could be a glandular problem." Well, our endocrine glands *are* a major player in metabolism and weight management, and can contribute to obesity. But did you know that more often our glands develop functional disorders from toxins and poisons in our food, air, water, and from living in our polluted world?

That's right—toxins are making us fat! Consider the following:

- Some toxins, like bisphenol-A from plastics and atrazine from herbicides, mimic estrogen. What does estrogen do? It helps cells grow and divide faster, and an excess can make you fat.

- Many cattle farmers feed estrogen to their cows in order to fatten them up quickly and economically. When we eat beef and drink milk, guess what? We fatten up too!

- Heavy metals like mercury cause pituitary malfunction. When the pituitary gland suffers, it can't send the proper messages to the thyroid gland. And when the thyroid gland suffers, our metabolisms go awry.

- Perchlorate, a rocket fuel chemical frequently found in our water supply, and fluoride are also thyroid suppressants that affect our metabolism—and not for the better!

- Food chemicals and chemicals in drinks can add to weight gain and cellular stress. **The flavor enhancer monosodium glutamate (MSG) is believed to be addictive and makes us crave the foods that make us gain weight**. Aspartame, which is added to sugarless foods, has recently been the focus of litigation because of its neurotoxic properties. Aspartame is often used in so-called "diet" foods, but the average weight loss when aspartame consumption is stopped is eight pounds. How ironic!

Let's talk about weight gain and our brains. Is there a connection? You bet! We've already learned that the brain acts as a sponge for chemicals. How? Well, chemicals are fat-soluble and are stored in fat cells. The brain, which is composed of two-thirds fat, becomes a dumping ground for unhealthy chemicals. Makes sense, doesn't it?

And it probably also comes as no surprise that this has terrible consequences. With so many chemicals in our world today, our neurotransmitter levels can suffer, creating cravings to attempt to restore the proper levels to our brains. Some addiction specialists believe addictions of many types are the body's attempt to restore the ideal levels of neurotransmitters in the brain. Just think of the millions of Americans today who seek relief from weight gain, fatigue, anxiety, and depression through prescription drugs designed to balance brain chemistry.

Let's also talk about weight control and adrenal function. Wondering where your adrenal glands are? Well, you have two, and each one sits atop each of your kidneys. These glands might be small, but they are powerful too! Healthy adrenals improve digestion, burn fat more efficiently, and give the body strength throughout the day. **The adrenal's role in fat burning is through their production of adrenaline and noradrenalin, which cause the breakdown and release of fat into energy**. When our adrenal glands are overworked, we often feel tired. What makes our adrenal glands work too hard? Things like stress, too much sugar, not enough rest, and processing toxic chemicals. And overworked adrenal glands often go hand-in-hand with a sluggish thyroid. So what do we do when we are feeling tired? We reach for a quick fix, namely food that will give us energy. But often these foods are bad for us. They are loaded with carbs, sugar, caffeine, and are fattening.

Another thing about adrenal glands-- trying to lose weight while suffering from adrenal overload and toxicity is almost impossible. Without adrenal power, our fat-burning ability is

greatly reduced, and for many this reason alone is why diets fail. Furthermore, trying to adhere to an exercise regime is a huge challenge when our adrenals carry a toxic burden and have suffered decades of stress.

What *else* is making us fat? Well, let's talk about how we treat our digestive systems in general. I think this is important because the digestive system is an area where major weight loss barriers can be found. Why? Well, many of us eat foods we shouldn't, namely foods we are allergic to or sensitive to. These allergies, or sensitivities, can lead to inflammation, bloating, and indigestion. And oddly enough, for whatever reason we actually *crave* the foods we are allergic or sensitive to. Let's take dairy products as an example. They contain a chemical called casein, which is thought to have an effect similar to morphine on the brain. So what happens after we eat dairy products? **We *crave* still more milk, cheese, ice cream, and other foods containing casein. But how about this fact? Casein is used as carpenter's glue and is also the adhesive used on beer bottle labels. Does it glue up your cells as well? Most likely!**

But before we go there, let's talk bout another source of disharmony that can contribute to unwanted weight gain. The hypothalamus and pituitary glands. The hypothalamus, located at the base of the brain, regulates the network of glands along the nervous system and the pituitary gland. The hypothalamus also regulates hunger and body temperature in the body. The pituitary, when healthy, protects us from fatigue due to excessive mental stress, along with many other functions. It also relays messages to the thyroid gland. When the pituitary is the problem, prescription drugs to boost the thyroid overlook the actual underlying problem and serve only to cover up the symptoms. Both the hypothalamus and pituitary are areas of toxin accumulation and therefore abnormal function can occur from various toxins and contribute to obesity.

Parasites also wreak havoc with our digestive systems. That's right—parasites! Parasites have been in the news recently as a factor in weight management. Dr. Robert O. Young, in the magazine *First for Women* (October 2006), suggests that "the natural by-products of parasites are acids that make 32% of the women in the U.S. sick, tired, and fat." He also states, "The body's self-preservation system can make the problem worse by shuffling the acidic waste from parasites into the fat cells and slowing metabolic rate, so more protective fat must be stored. This is the body's way of getting acids out of circulation, but it makes losing weight virtually impossible."

When we have undigested food particles rotting in our digestive tract, those particles attract parasites. Just as buzzards and vultures in the wild will feed on the remains of dead animals, parasites enter and breed to attempt to "eat up the leftovers" and survive. Cleaning up the digestive tract discourages parasites from "setting up camp" in our gut. Yet many of us have had parasitic infestations for so many years, dietary changes alone will not suffice in many cases. What's the answer? Don't worry, I'll tell you how to handle parasites, which may be your roadblock to weight loss, a bit later.

Toxicity to our insulin receptors is another reason we might be getting fat. Insulin receptors, which are found on the surface cells throughout the body, can stop responding to insulin and cause a condition called *insulin resistance*. With insulin resistance, insulin and blood glucose levels can be high, yet the cells are starving for glucose, which causes sugar cravings, overeating, and weight gain.

And guess what? These insulin receptors are also vulnerable to environmental chemicals, heavy metals, saturated fats, and food toxins such as MSG. As a matter of fact, studies have confirmed that MSG alone causes gross obesity in animals. And most processed food contains significant amounts of MSG.

The incidence of Type II diabetes has increased some 600% over the last 30 years. Historically a disease of overweight, middle-aged people, it is not unusual today to see children as young as ten who have developed this devastating disorder. Many theories have attempted to explain why we are now seeing such an explosion of Type II diabetes, but none really meet all the observations associated with the condition. One probable factor is the huge amount of MSG and excitotoxic food additives consumed today. The amount of these food additives has doubled every decade since their introduction in 1948.

If healthier eating alone could make overweight people lose weight, we'd see a lot more permanent weight loss. Many people have failed multiple times when attempting to lose weight, and do not want to succumb to failure once more. **But very frequently, *their real failure was overlooking the true underlying causes of their metabolic dysfunction*.** Sadly, most medical doctors are *not* trained in looking for these hidden factors, which can be lifelong barriers to weight loss when ignored.

Chemicals That Damage the Thyroid

- Plastics
- Solvents
- Synthetic rubber
- Metals
- Mycotoxins
- Prescription Drugs
- Environmental pollutants
- Food additives, dyes, and preservatives
- Halogens (bromine, chlorine, and fluoride)
- Growth hormones
- Pesticides

CHAPTER 8

THE GAS PEDAL FOR ACCELERATED AGING

Whoa! Let's Slow Down Aging
Slowing Down the Aging Clock

You've seen the effects of oxidative stress many times--wrinkles, sagging skin, and age spots are some of the obvious *external* indica-tors. This accelerated aging process occurs not just on the *outside*, but within every cell in the body. The same process of oxidation takes place when you cut an apple and it turns brown and when your jewelry tarnishes and when iron develops rust.

Stress Running Out of Control

When the process of oxidation occurs faster than our bodies can *repair the damage*, breakdown happens at the sites most damaged. Serious degenerative disease results because oxidative stress was allowed to go unchecked over too long a period of time.

How Toxins Oxidize Us & Cause Damage

Inside every cell of the body is a tiny power plant, called the *mito-chondria*. As this power plant uses the oxygen we inhale to create energy, sometimes an unstable molecule is created, called a *free radical*. "When these dangerous free radicals are not quickly neutralized by an anti-oxidant they can go on to create more volatile free radicals, damaging cell walls, vessel walls, proteins, fats, and even the DNA nucleus of our cells. This reaction has been shown to actually create bursts of light within our bodies!"

"When hazardous free radicals penetrate into the DNA of a cell, they damage its "blueprint" so that the cell will produce mutated cells that can then replicate without the normal controls." The most obvious manifestation of mutated cells growing out of control is cancer.

"Imagine yourself sitting in front of a crackling fireplace…the fires burns safely and beautifully most of the time, but on occasion, out pops a hot cinder that lands on your carpet and burns a hole in it. One cinder by itself doesn't pose much of a threat…..but if this sparking and popping continues month after month, year after year, you have a pretty 'ratty' carpet in front of your fireplace. So, the fireplace represents the tiny power plant of the cell (the mitochondria) and the hot cinder is the dangerous free radical, and the carpet is your body. Whichever part of your body receives the most free radical damage will be the first to wear out and potentially cause one of these degenerative diseases. If it's your arteries, you could have a heart attack or stroke. If it's your brain, you could develop Alzheimer's dementia or Parkinson's disease, memory loss or brain fog. If it's your joints, you could develop arthritis."

The Toxic Perpetrators of Oxidative Stress

Now you understand more about toxins and how they cause oxidative stress, and are a direct assault on the well-being and functioning of cells, tissues, glands and organs. This on-going 'war' may not *always* result in degenerative disease; it may aggravate an existing condition or cause a disorder in the proper function of a body system, gland or organ.

Toxins such as perchlorate or fluoride causing oxidative stress in the thyroid, for example, may cause a sluggish thyroid, or hypothyroidism. You may recall from an earlier chapter how lead can affect the brain, lowering IQ. Oxidative stress caused by toxins in the joints may cause an old injury to flare up again. *Toxins invade every cell, organ and gland in the body, creating oxidative stress, dysfunction and havoc.* This is why a whole body detoxification is far superior and more effective than a mere colon cleanse or liver cleanse, which only address those specific organs.

In addition to food additives and preservatives, and pesticides in our foods which all cause oxidative stress, some foods themselves are major sources of free radicals. Processed oils and highly heated oils and foods made with them are prime perpetrators. Most snack chips and commercial baked goods are made with harmful fats. Better oils include cold-pressed olive oil, grapeseed oil, coconut oil and organic butter.

"Excessive sugar intake can also contribute to free radical damage. White and brown sugars, and even sugar from so-called natural sources, such as fruit juices, maple syrup and honey get converted into triglycerides by the liver and are subject to free radical damage. These damaged fats then promptly attack your arteries and directly contribute to cardiovascular disease. **Additionally, cancer and tumor cells feed off sugar."**

Anti-Oxidants: Your "Ammunition" against Oxidative Stress

The *good news* is that you can fight the accelerated aging process and offset oxidative stress with ammunition called *anti-oxidants.*

"Recall the analogy of the fireplace (your cell's power plant) with the hot cinders (free radicals) popping? Damaging the carpet (your body)?

Anti-oxidants are like the glass doors or fine wire mesh we place in front of our fireplace. *The sparks are still going to fly, but our carpet will then be protected."*

So the goal is to provide the body with adequate protection in the form of good nutrition. If 'eating a balanced diet' were enough-- we wouldn't be seeing degenerative disease running rampant as it is today. This is why in addition to wholesome organic foods, we require nutritional supplements. **How do we assess *how much* oxidative stress is happening in the body? Using frequency testing, we check for specific biomarkers which indicate oxidative stress.** When our fats (including the brain) are under oxidative stress, a marker called MDA tests positive. When our proteins are under attack and losing the battle, a marker called NT shows up. With damage to the DNA and RNA, markers known as 8-OHd G and 8-OHG are present. The more biomarkers present, the worse the oxidative stress and damage to the cells.

Our 'super-allies' in the battle against oxidative stress include specific vitamins, minerals, enzymes, herbal formulas and oils. And just as with foods, all supplements are *not* created equal. Quite often people come to us for help who may have been taking high-quality supplements, but not at the best dose for their needs, as well as omitting some nutrients crucial in creating *lasting changes in health.* **This is why working with a qualified expert in targeted nutrition is the key to protecting your health. Individual nutritional needs are as unique as your fingerprints.** In addition to performing nutritional analysis testing, other factors we consider are a person's health history, diet, occupation, activity level, stress level, current health status, use of prescribed medicines, over-the-counter medicines, and their personal preference for taking supplements in capsule and tablet form or in liquid form.

By assisting the body to clean up and eliminate the *cause* of oxidative stress and then the pathways of detoxification (liver, colon, kidneys, lungs, lymph, skin) and providing the highest-quality supplements as 'ammunition' to assist in repair and re-building.......health can often be fully regained! Your body has innate God-given healing power; when the toxic burden is lifted and cells have what they *need* to do their jobs, the stage is set for healing to happen!

I cannot emphasize enough the importance of detoxification as the 1st step to re-building a healthier happier you. Many well-meaning friends, associates, health-food store employees, and popular magazines offer advice on taking this-or-that supplement for specific ailments....but when toxins are the underlying *cause* of malfunction (and they usually are) you may be just taking supplements that cover-up symptoms and *not be addressing the root of the problem.* **Your good health is your most valuable possession....isn't it worthy of special care and attention?**

<u>ANTI-OXIDANTS</u>

Alpha lipoic acid
Beta carotene
Bioflavonoid
Catechins / quercetins
Cholesterol
Co-Q10
Curcumin
Enzymes
Green tea
Glutathione
Herbal compounds & foods
Melatonin
N-acetyl cysteine (NAC)
Resveratrol
Selenium
Super oxide dismutase (SOD)
Various phyto-chemicals
Vitamin A
Vitamin C
Vitamin E
Zinc

TOXINS CAUSING OXIDATIVE STRESS

Additives / preservatives in food
Alcohol
Bad fats / oils
Chemicals
Chlorinated water
Cigarette smoke
Cleaning fluids / products
Drugs
Emotional stress
Food colorings / dyes
Heavy metals
Pesticides
Physical stress
Poor diet
Radiation
Smog
Solvents
Sugars
EMF

CHAPTER 9

ARE YOU ALWAYS TIRED AND EXHAUSTED?

Put Pizazz Back Into Your Life!
No Spunk in Your Trunk?

> *"For most of my life, I've not felt good. I've always been tired; my mother called me a hypochondriac because the medical doctors couldn't find anything wrong. Finally they said it was fibromyalgia and sleep problems. My medical doctor wasn't able to help the fibromyalgia pain. I was fed up and tired of taking anti-depressants.*
>
> *"Now my energy is much better and my joints feel much better. The baker's cyst in the back of my knee is reduced; the MD had told me surgery was the only thing that would help it. In the past, whenever I'd paint my toes, my calves would have severe cramps. It's now completely gone in my left leg and almost gone in my right leg.*
>
> *"I'm just really pleased and I'm only halfway through (detoxification). When you finally don't feel so bad anymore, the snowball stops rolling down the hill and begins to melt.*

I don't remember EVER feeling this good before! Now I feel like walking, exercising, and painting a room. I've already told others about Nutrition Wellness Center.
—Taffar
Palm Harbor, Florida

"Since childhood I always felt tired, suffered from migraine headaches and had pain somewhere everyday. As I grew older I developed severe menstrual cramps and depression. My health became progressively worse in the past 10 to 15 years. I was diagnosed with chronic fatigue and fibromyalgia. It got so bad I couldn't work, take care of the family or myself for that matter. I literally stayed on the couch and felt "dead inside."

"I went to all kinds of doctors, who ran all kinds of diagnostics and prescribed multiple drugs. I still couldn't get off the couch and yet I was prescribed more pills.

"I first heard about Nutrition Wellness Center from Frank M. and his wife Robin. He had devastating health issues over a year ago. I saw the difference in him and hoped Dr Martin could help me.

"Since doing Dr. Martin's program I don't have the "fatigue" anymore, just a normal tired. I have a strong desire

to do things like laundry, working in the garden, planting trees, or shopping. I feel organized. My mother says I look much better, and more healthy. My friends comment my skin looks nice and my eyes have brightness to them. Even my massage therapist noticed my muscles are looser and less tight. Keith, my husband, loves having me go out with him on field service calls. I feel like doing that now.

"I have learned so much more in the past 2 months. I had a lot of the pieces to the puzzle and Dr Martin and his staff helped me put it all together. I am so impressed with the great support system there especially since they teach the very ideas that form the foundation of my belief system regarding healthcare. I act on my convictions and I would absolutely recommend Nutrition Wellness Center to others. I have tried so many other things and it would work for 2-3 weeks then fail. I know I am getting better and this time is going to work. When I first came to Nutrition Wellness Center I was in despair. Now I feel happy with the results and relieved."

—Sharren

Vero Beach, FL

Face it, we live our lives at a much more hectic pace than we used to. We are busier than ever juggling work, home, children, and our interests. It is no wonder we are a little tired; that our energy feels not quite up to par.

However, for some people, the fatigue is crushing. And I'm not talking about ordering pizza because the day was so hectic that you are too tired to make dinner. I'm talking about the kind of fatigue that makes it hard for you to get out of bed, let alone function at home or at work.

This is the type of fatigue that can turn a previously active life upside down.

It wasn't that long ago when doctors were hesitant to name this condition. It was a nebulous illness at best, with no type of test or markers to determine what was causing it. Today doctors call this illness *Chronic Fatigue Syndrome*, (CFS) or sometimes *Myalgic Encephalomyelitis*.

What is Chronic Fatigue Syndrome? Well, in addition to life-altering fatigue, other symptoms include neurological problems, sleep issues, headaches, sore and aching muscles and joints, and a sore throat. It usually strikes people between the ages of 20 and 40, and can last anywhere from a few months to years.

So what do chemicals have to do with Chronic Fatigue Syndrome? It appears they play a very prominent role. We already know that chemicals damage many parts of the body—the brain, nerves, hormones, glands, and organs. And guess what? Every single one of these body parts is integral in the production of energy and activity. So when chemicals damage these body parts, it just makes sense that our energy and activity levels are directly affected.

As I mentioned before, Chronic Fatigue Syndrome is a fairly new disease. It's interesting to note that as the manufacture of chemicals and toxins reaches an all-time high, so do the symptoms associated with Chronic Fatigue Syndrome.

The direct effect of oxidation on glands and the brain can lead to Chronic Fatigue Syndrome. Interruption of brain chemistry, thyroid and adrenal function can contribute to the growing affliction of Chronic Fatigue Syndrome. The indirect effect of toxins (as discussed in Chapter 5) is the other part of the equation.

Veterans of the first Gulf War who were exposed to chemicals have a much higher rate of Chronic Fatigue Syndrome than those vets who were not, which tells us something. So does the fact that a recent study showed farmers exposed to organophosphates, such as those used in sheep dip, had a higher degree of fatigue-related illnesses.

Metals, as well, affect the nerves, hormone, and immune systems, all of which are related to energy. So it comes as no surprise that people determined to have mercury, nickel, or cadmium in their systems often suffer from lack of energy or go on to develop Chronic Fatigue Syndrome.

But whether you notice a lack of energy or suffer from Chronic Fatigue Syndrome, all is not lost. Once the issues of toxins and chemicals are addressed, a good individualized detox program, combined with avoiding certain chemicals, can restore your energy and vitality.

**Toxins Associated with Fatigue and
Chronic Fatigue Syndrome**

- Toxic metals
- Pesticides
- Organochlorines
- Solvents
- Halogens
- Plastics
- Certain prescribed drugs

CHAPTER 10

TOXINS AND DIGESTIVE PROBLEMS

Eating Better Easier
Getting Ahead of Gut Problems

"The irritable bowel syndrome. I have no problem with my stomach anymore. When the MD saw me today, I used to have 18 tender points. Now I just have 14.

"I'm no longer bed-ridden on my bad days. I've been able to cut way down on the Imitrex (medicine for chronic daily migraines).

"My MD, a pain management doctor, said he'll refer other patients to Nutrition Wellness Center, because he's so pleased with what's happening. My internist also agreed this program seems to be working.

"I have no trouble with my left knee now. I used to not be able to walk some days."

—Barbara
Estero, Florida

We've all heard the saying a million times. You are what you eat! So if you suffer from bloating, indigestion, stomach pain, and inflammation, then the news probably isn't all that good, is it?

The truth is, there's a lot of information out there concerning diet. And most of us have paid attention and do our best to eat healthfully. We eat, or make a good effort to eat, the amount of fruits, veggies, and grains suggested to us.

But did you know that all those foods you think are good for you-- swordfish, strawberries, salmon, apples, and lettuce--can be damaging your digestive system?

If you are wondering how this can be, I do want to make sure you understand that the food itself, in its organic form, is not the problem here. It is more the side dish of chemicals, pollutants, pesticides, and herbicides that come along *with* these foods that are the *real* issue.

We already know how today's agriculture and chemicals go together like, well, peanut butter and jelly. When we eat food contaminated with toxins, our digestive systems are front and center when it comes to dealing with them. On a daily basis, our digestive systems are assaulted with metals, food additives, food preservatives, dyes and colorings, pesticides, herbicides, solvents, and other pollutants. Worse, our digestive systems don't stand up well to chemical damage at all. How do toxins damage the digestive system?

First of all, they damage the interior wall of the stomach, which make it difficult to absorb the nutrients, vitamins, and minerals that you need. On top of that, a digestive system that constantly comes into contact with toxic chemicals can result in an imbalance of digestive juices and hormones, which can result in undigested food or ulceration. Chemicals can also kill the good bacteria in the intestinal tract, which allows the *bad* bacteria to multiply and cause issues like infections and inflammation.

Other problems chemicals cause include damaging the parts of the brain and the hormones that control digestion, poisoning the immune system, affecting the muscle walls of the bowel, and exposing the digestive tract to carcinogens. When your digestive system is under a constant barrage of toxic chemicals, at some point it isn't going to be able to take it anymore. It's going to revolt!

It's interesting to note that food intolerances and allergies are on the rise. I don't remember "peanut-free" tables in my elementary school cafeteria, but you can't walk into a school now without encountering one. Lactose intolerance, while not life-threatening, is also on the rise.

So what's up? Scientists have devoted lots of studies asking why people are reacting to their food now more than ever before. **But here's my take on it. When you consider the amount of toxins we encounter on a daily basis, as well as what they do to our digestive systems, it's no wonder that people who are more exposed to chemical toxins like pesticides, solvents, air contaminants, and metals are reacting to foods they might otherwise tolerate. Toxic chemicals promote food sensitivity and allergies by both damaging the underlying immune system, and by directly triggering food intolerance reactions. When chemicals over stimulate the immune system, it overreacts to substances it normally wouldn't. Unfortunately, sometimes it overreacts to food.**

Another kind of food intolerance is directly related to the *chemicals in and around food*, and not really to the *foods themselves*. Examples would include preservatives, dyes, additives, and flavorings. Sensitivity to these things can certainly mimic true food allergies, but are different in that the sensitivity is related to the chemical, and not to the actual food.

Inflammatory Bowel Disease is another fairly new disease that is on the rise. The cause of IBD is unknown, and the medical community largely agrees that it is incurable. However, the medical community agrees on something else: a malfunctioning immune system plays a significant role in the disease. So you see where I'm going here, don't you? IBD is a hyperactive immune syndrome. And what makes your immune system overreact? That's right. Chemicals!

Chemicals That Can Trigger IBS

• Additives in carbonated drinks
• Chemicals found in tobacco products
• Fluoride
• Pollution
• Certain prescription medicines
• Solvents
• Food additives and preservatives
• Metals

Irritable Bowel Syndrome is another common complaint; in fact, one in five people in the United States have this condition. Symptoms include sudden urge to empty the bowels, indigestion, excess mucus, bloating, abdominal pain, gas, diarrhea, and constipation.

What role do toxic chemicals play in IBS? Well, we've already determined that our digestive systems often can't handle the onslaught of chemicals they face. Remember, the intestines are directly exposed to any toxic chemicals that enter our bodies through food. Too many toxic chemicals affect the nerves, mineral levels and overall body pH that determine how and when the bowel muscle contracts and expands are affected. The toxic chemicals can damage all of these factors that control the bowel, and the result can be IBS.

Okay, enough of all that bad news! The *good news* is that digestive problems linked to toxic chemicals can be managed, sometimes even cured. The goal is to add a detox and nutrition program to your life that will ensure the immune system doesn't go into overdrive. When the immune system is under control, the digestive system will be less sensitive and less likely to flare up.

CHAPTER 11

ANXIETY AND DEPRESSION

De-Bugging Your Brain
Fixing Glitches in Your Super-Computer-
Your BRAIN!

> *"My medical doctor wanted me to have a liver biopsy since my liver enzymes were really bad. I told my gastroenterologists' assistant that I wanted to do a natural approach through Dr. Martin's office instead. My first nutritional test at Nutrition Wellness Center was less than four months ago. My primary MD sent me back for blood work recently; my cholesterol had been 275, its 203 now. All my liver enzymes and blood work were normal. My medical doctor said whatever I'm doing to keep it up since its working.*
>
> *"I have no more brain fogginess. I used to have it all the time. In school when I was studying to be an esthetician, it was difficult. My thinking is much clearer now; and no more*

mood swings. I also don't have irritable bowel syndrome anymore. I'm not nearly as tired now. And I'm less bloated. I used to have more fat around the middle. Now I don't have it.

"My husband, who was skeptical at first, said he can tell a world of difference in the way I look and the way I feel."
—Sharon
Sarasota, Florida

What's up with all the brain-related diseases and disorders that have cropped up? Is something literally poisoning our minds? Quite possibly.

It would be convenient to blame the rise of brain-related diseases and disorders on an aging population, but the fact is these types of diseases are cropping up at earlier and earlier ages. Take autism, for example, which is seen more today in children than ever before. Could our brain-related diseases and disorders have something to do with the environments in which we live?

Well, consider this fact. Twenty five percent of the chemicals in our environment are known neurotoxins. And in case you are wondering, a neurotoxin is a toxin that poisons our nerves. **Our children are experiencing an onslaught of these chemicals, and their brains are just developing. It is no wonder that developmental brain disorders are on the rise.**

Let's spend a little time talking about what makes our nervous systems so sensitive to chemical toxins. The brain has an excellent blood supply, and is also made up of fatty tissue. And these things are great . . . they help our brains control our bodies. **But the good blood supply and the fatty tissue means that toxins have no trouble getting to the brain, and once there they take up residence in the fat. Our brains literally soak up the toxins that we encounter in our environment.**

Once these toxins have taken up residence in the brain they can be pretty hard to remove. One reason is that there isn't enough antioxidant nutrients present in the brain to neutralize the free radicals that are a result of the chemicals. Add to this the fact that nerve cells are somewhat delicate and don't regenerate well, and you can see how toxic chemicals contribute to brain diseases. Brain diseases that are more common today than ever before include Parkinson's, Alzheimer's, ADHD, Autism, and Multiple Sclerosis.

Statistics today indicate 1 out of every 150 children born today will be Autistic. To me, that is pretty scary statistics and should be a big wake-up call to action.

Mood disturbances are a common problem these days. Just consider the number of prescription drugs out there on the market designed to beat the blues or lift anxiety. Why do so many people suffer from anxiety and depression? Well, the times we live in are stressful, that's certain. But our exposure to toxic chemicals, combined with fewer mood stabilizing nutrients as a result of our processed, less healthy diets, makes it not all that surprising that mood issues are on the rise.

Depression, anxiety, and other mood-related disorders are said to be caused by imbalances in the levels of mood-enhancing natural substances called neurotransmitters. In a nutshell, these are the things that keep us smiling! There's a whole host of prescription drugs out there designed to boost our neurotransmitters.

But wait a second. Do we really need prescription drugs to boost our neurotransmitters? When you consider that 90% of the toxic chemicals we encounter affect our neurotransmitters, perhaps the key to happiness is less in a prescription drug and more in managing the toxins in our life.

The major villains that wreak havoc on our neurotransmitters include many different kinds of prescription drugs, pesticides, environmental pollutants, solvents, and metals. As a matter of fact, a study showed that removing mercury fillings improved the moods of 70% of those who suffered from mercury-related illnesses, including depression. Those who work in the chemical industry are more prone to depression than those who are not, but even those of us out in the mainstream are exposed to mood-altering toxins such as pesticides, solvents, and prescription drugs. Who knew that spraying a little DEET on your skin to banish the bugs on a hot summer night would also banish the happy hormones from your brain?

But as I mentioned before, you don't necessarily need drugs to get rid of the blues. The goal, instead, should be to lower your body burden of toxins by going on an individually designed detoxification plan, limiting your future contact with toxins, and making sure you get the right nutrients to your brain to boost those happy hormones!

Another toxin-related brain issue is more nebulous and harder to pin a name on. As a matter of fact, if this disorder had a name, we might forget it! Some of us attribute this condition to our busy lives and always being on the run. I call it brain fog, and I say that toxins play a part!

We've all forgotten someone's name, neglected to run an important errand, or lost our keys at one time or another. But for some people forgetfulness, the inability to focus, spaciness, and confusion are an everyday way of life. But unfortunately, memory loss, unless it morphs into dementia, is not treated as a real issue by the medical community. It is often shrugged off and neglected to be treated as a "real" problem. We live in a world of band-aiding the symptoms versus addressing the cause.

In fact, there are a lot of toxins known to have a negative effect on memory. Consider that many pesticides were developed during World War II as nerve agents and you'll see what I mean. Pesticides work by poisoning the pest by rapidly paralyzing it so it quickly stops breathing and moving. And these pesticides are now often found in our food supply. So what effect do you think they have on us? After all, are we really all that different from bugs? We both have nervous systems, right?

Metals and solvents are two additional types of toxins known to affect memory. The goal of restoring your memory can be met with the right detox program, good nutrition, and the avoidance of toxins in the future. Chapter 11 describes much more about toxins and the brain and the havoc that can happen when toxins build up in our 'super-computer'.

CHAPTER 12

CANCER

How NOT to Grow Cancer Cells

Cancer is one of our most dreaded diseases. First of all, curing it, assuming you have the type of cancer that can be cured, is a battle. Second of all, conventional medical treatment for cancer is often poisonous, and the result is that the cure is almost as bad as the disease.

But there's no doubt about it, more and more people are developing cancer despite our efforts to ward it off with things like screenings, diet, and a whole host of protective measures designed to ensure that we don't get cancer in the first place. Unfortunately, more than one million people per year are diagnosed with cancer, and about half of them will succumb to the disease.

What exactly is cancer? Cancer happens when something damages our normal cells, which makes them divide uncontrollably. Things that cause cancer are called carcinogens. And what makes it on to the list of carcinogens? Well, you've come this far, so you've probably guessed . . . *many* of the chemicals we encounter on a daily basis.

And beware. The list is long! Pesticides, metals, environmental pollutants, plastics, fluoride, solvents, synthetic steroids, and artificial growth hormones are all on the list of possible suspects.

I hate to paint an even scarier picture, but of the 70,000 or so chemicals that you or I might run into during our daily lives, do you know how many have actually been tested as carcinogens? About 300. And of those 300, about half have been shown to cause cancer in animals. I think we all assume that just because something is available commercially for consumer use it has been tested and is safe. Unfortunately, that's just not the case. The fact remains that the majority of chemicals we encounter on a day-to-day basis have *never been tested* to see whether they are cancer causing. Based on the testing that has been carried out, we can only guess at the results.

The most common cancers that occur as a result of toxic chemicals include breast, brain, prostate, urinary tract, and lymphomas and leukemia's. Furthermore, chemicals can spur on the *growth* of cancer in general, making it harder to contain or cure once it has been diagnosed.

Toxins that can Cause Cancer

- Chlorine
- Detergents
- Alcohols
- Pesticides
- Organochlorines
- Plastics
- Solvents
- Synthetic estrogen
- Metals
- Mycotoxins

The good news, if there can be good news with cancer, is that being aware that chemicals cause cancer can help you defend yourself against cancer, as well as fight back if you already have it. A target specific designed detoxification, nutritional, and chemical avoidance program can not only put the odds in your favor of not getting cancer in the first place, it can also help your body fight cancer.

The National Cancer Institute website states that 85% of all cancers come from environmental toxins, diet and lifestyle. Detoxification and nutritional support is not a treatment for cancer, but a common sense approach to help create the optimal environment for healing and recovery with conventional medical treatment.

CHAPTER 13

ALLERGIES?

Relief at LAST!

> *"Since starting my detoxification program at Nutrition Wellness Center the pain in my face is 75% better in less than one month. I've had this facial pain for 20 years. It hurt so bad I couldn't even touch my eyelashes; now I can. Before, when the weather would change, the facial pain was horrible. Now I don't react to weather changes.*
>
> *"They'd (MDs) been giving me Tegretol, a seizure drug. It made me a zombie. I wasn't able to drive taking it and it didn't help the facial pain. Then the MDs told me surgery to cut the facial nerve in my face was my only choice. My face would have sagged as if I'd had a stroke.*
>
> *"I used to have very dark circles under my eyes. I was so tired. Now I feel a lot better. I get up and I'm not as tired and I have the energy to go to work. I don't need allergy shots anymore. My skin is getting better. My mind is so clear. I'm so happy!"*
>
> —Angela
> Sarasota, Florida

Many studies show that toxic chemicals damage our immune system. And when our immune system is damaged, we overreact to things that bodies normally should handle. Whether our bodies overreact by breaking out into hives our by having itchy eyes and runny noses, we call it the same thing: allergies.

Pesticides, environmental pollutants, toxic metals, solvents, plastics, and other chemicals destroy our immune systems. When our immune system isn't functioning properly it does one of two things: it either underreacts, causing susceptibility to disease and infection, or it over-reacts, causing allergic reactions like hives, runny nose and eyes, sneezing, wheezing, and in the worst cases, anaphylactic shock.

Lots of people suffer from allergies. And most people can figure out what they are allergic to based on when they react and what substances they have been in contact with. How do most medical doctors deal with allergies? In most cases, the patient is instructed to avoid the allergen, and may even be put on an anti-histamine or other drug to control symptoms. Unfortunately, while this course of action treats the symptoms, it does *not* treat the underlying causes. To make matters worse, some allergens, like trees, are almost im-possible to avoid. And the drugs designed to combat allergies rarely if ever relieve patients of all symptoms. Many also have side effects that make the patient tired, or hyperactive.

Let's talk about how chemicals put our bodies into overdrive. Metals, for example, like mercury and aluminum, put into action those im-mune system cells that are designed to fight unwanted intruders. Your immune system is poised and ready to fight! Cytokines, which are basically your cells' fighting weapons, are built up, which am-plify the cells' fight. So what happens? The allergic reaction is even more severe. In a nutshell, chemicals give our cells weapons and get them all amped up to fight when there is really no need to.

Do you ever wonder why some allergies are developed later in life? When the chemicals tamper with our immune system, eventually our immune system has trouble differentiating between substances that *are* indeed harmful and those that *are not*. What happens is that when the chemical level in our bodies reaches a certain level—when our immune system gets heightened to a certain point—it fights, and begins to reject, substances it *used to* accept.

Chemical Substances Known to Trigger Allergies

- Cigarette smoke
- Chlorine
- Prescription and non-prescription drugs
- Fluoride
- Food preservatives, additives, and dyes
- Latex rubber
- Pesticides
- Solvents
- Plastics
- Toxic metals
- Toiletries
- Wood preservatives
- Environmental pollutants

While allergies such as food allergies, hay fever, allergic eczema, and hives can all be treated symptomatically, treating the *root of the problem* is the best way to go. Since allergies are caused by an out-of-whack immune system, the goal should be to rebalance the immune system by undergoing detoxification to rid the body of current chemicals, making lifestyle changes to avoid toxins in the future, and maintaining a good nutrition and supplement program to keep the immune system functioning as it is intended.

"I have to admit I was brought kicking and screaming and full of skepticism, by my sisters Caroline and Susan, to see you. I naturally thought there was nothing wrong with me, as I've always been healthy as a horse.

"For having nothing wrong, you have made my Spring and Fall pollen, animal, and mold allergies disappear. My sinus clears up to where I can talk without hoarseness for the first time in years. You've cured me of dizziness, and have made my insides clear of parasites, dyes, pesticides, chemicals, metals, and most bacteria. You have made growing cataracts in my eyes reverse to just a trace, and have taken my cholesterol from 275 to 220.

"How fortunate for me to have such a short list. I see folks who are suffering so much and come great distances for your help and knowledge. How fortunate for me to live close enough to run down on a regular basis for preventative maintenance. How fortunate for me that my skepticism has been replaced with genuine gratitude and respect for your abilities.

"Now, about my 63-year-old back... Just fix it one more time and I promise not to move my clients' furniture from one room to another, to love my grandchildren without picking them up, to assign digging in my rose bed to a young neighbor across the street, and to not jump on the trampoline, ski, or skate anymore. I'll try to be good in this respect.

"I am very grateful and thankful to you, and for the patience and efficiency of your wonderful staff."

—Margaret

Sarasota, Florida

CHAPTER 14

AUTO-IMMUNE

You CAN Re-Set Your Immune Response

"I can walk, I can move my fingers. My finger that was so swollen and arthritic is normal again and I can wear my rings. The large lump on the back of my neck is gone. My spine was swollen and the huge bump on the back of my right leg is gone. I was in a wheelchair from a chemotherapy drug called Methotrexate, given to me for rheumatoid arthritis, or scleroderma, they weren't sure which. On the steroid drug, I had gained 127 pounds . . . and on Dr. Martin's program I lost it all and more. The drugs had made my hair thin, dull, and it was falling out. I had several bald spots. Now my hair is thick and shiny and people say I glow.

"Everyone I've sent to the Nutrition Wellness Center looks better after doing your program.

"My medical doctor said he's definitely seen a miracle and that I would have been dead had I not gone to the Nutrition Wellness Center."

—Kathy

Danby, Vermont

As long as we are talking about our immune systems and how they can sometimes fail to differentiate between foreign invaders and harmless substances, let's talk about autoimmune diseases.

Autoimmune diseases work very similar to allergies, but instead of the body being allergic to something like food, trees, or something we come into contact with, the body fights its *own* tissues it is designed to protect.

Imagine a heightened immune system unleashing its full fury against its own body tissues, and you can see how debilitating and sometimes even deadly, autoimmune disorders can be. Your immune system actually sees your own tissues as the enemy, and will not stop until it has destroyed them.

Autoimmune disorders are affecting more and more people. Diseases such as rheumatoid arthritis, juvenile diabetes, ankylosing spondylitis, lupus, scleroderma, Hashimoto's Thyroiditis and Addison's disease are much more prevalent today than they were at the turn of the century. Heredity does play a role in autoimmune diseases, but more and more people without a genetic link to these disorders are experiencing them. The link between chemicals and the increase in autoimmune diseases has been noted in several studies, most of which show that people in certain jobs, who are exposed to certain chemicals, have a greater incidence of autoimmune disorders.

How do chemicals trigger autoimmune disorders? In much the same way they do allergies. Basically, once the toxic body burden reaches a certain height, the level of immune system activity is increased. The immune system eventually has trouble discerning between friend and foe, so it produces what is called autoantibodies. Autoantibodies cause our own tissues to be labeled as foreign tissues, and when this happens our immune system attacks the very tissues it is designed to protect.

Unfortunately, once this process is set in motion your immune system won't stop until it accomplishes its goal. Because of this, autoimmune diseases are considered incurable. However, the immune system, and the reaction it has, can be soothed by ridding the body of toxic chemicals. If the autoimmune reaction is the result of toxic insult, a specific targeted detoxification and nutritional program is very beneficial. There are also some excellent herbal formulas that are effective in reducing the autoimmune reactions.

Chemicals That Can Trigger Autoimmune Diseases

- Pesticides
- Oral contraceptives
- Estrogen replacement therapy
- PCB's and PAH's
- Solvents
- Heavy metals, specifically mercury, gold and arsenic
- Hair products that contain aromatic amines
- Drugs that contain aromatic amines

CHAPTER 15

HIGH BLOOD PRESSURE & HEART DISEASE

Address the CAUSE, and Create the Solution!

> *"I had been on medication for my high triglyceride and high cholesterol levels. I was over-medicated. The medicine was harmful and my triglyceride and cholesterol levels didn't change. I heard about Nutrition Wellness Center through friends of our family—the three of them go there to see Dr. Martin. I came to Dr. Martin to manage my high blood pressure, to lose weight, to better my life, and to get out of some old habits. My high blood pressure and extra weight interfered with my attitude; mostly I was depressed and slept a lot.*
>
> *"Since coming to Nutrition Wellness Center, my triglyceride and cholesterol levels are good. My blood pressure is now 120/70 and it hadn't been that good for two or three years. My wife and I now follow the Diet and the nutritional program from Dr. Martin. I can see the results in*

the mirror. Even my complexion is better. I've lost 17 pounds; my previously 40-inch waist is now 36 inches. I have more energy—now I feel like going out and doing things.

"When I first came here (Nutrition Wellness Center) I wasn't sure . . . I've always been one you have to 'show me,' I'm not going to take your word for it. It was a journey; but I'm a believer now. 150%. Even my medical doctor is very happy with me being on Dr. Martin's program.

"My whole family in Tampa and Clearwater has noticed the positive changes—I'm more talkative and friendly, my fuse isn't as short now. My whole personality is back again after 20 years. My life has changed so much for the better. Everybody I've told about Nutrition Wellness Center, I've told them this was the BEST money I've ever spent."

—Doug

Northport, Florida

At the turn of the century, heart attacks were considered somewhat rare. Today, one out of two people will die from a heart-related condition. That's right, you read that stat correctly: *one out of two*!

The increase in heart disease is directly linked to our diet, lifestyles, and environment.

It makes sense that the increase in the amount of toxic chemicals we are exposed to would have an impact on our hearts. After all, our hearts are governed by hormones and nerves and are made up of muscle tissue. And we already know how these things are negatively impacted by the chemicals we encounter.

While you don't often turn on the evening news and hear about how toxic chemicals are contributing to our nation's growing heart disease, several studies *have* been done that link heart disease to certain chemicals. For example, industrial workers and cleaners who use chemicals are at a higher risk for cardiovascular disease than those who don't. Further studies have shown that exposure to toxic metals is connected to high blood pressure, and diabetes and high cholesterol are linked with increased levels of pesticides and environmental pollutants.

It's interesting to note that as cardiovascular disease increases, reasons are studied and new drugs are brought on to the market. Suffice it to say, the medical community has spent lots and lots of money trying to lessen the impact of cardiovascular disease on our society. Time and countless dollars have been spent trying to prevent, and also trying to cure, the heart diseases that are afflicting us.

How are chemicals linked to heart disease? First of all, chemicals can poison the heart tissues. Second, prolonged exposure to chemicals increases risk factors.

We already noted that the nerves play a large part in the functioning of the heart. And we know chemicals affect the nerves. In addition to the nerves, the other parts of the heart that are most sensitive to direct chemical exposure are the heart cells that control the heart beat, and the coronary arteries. When these areas are affected by chemicals, things such as heart arrhythmias, angina, and heart attack can follow.

The heart's long-term exposure to chemicals is more likely to result in diseases and disorders that affect the heart, such as high cholesterol, diabetes, and high blood pressure.

Chemicals That Can Trigger Heart Disease:

• Sulphur dioxide (also known as air pollution)
• Chlorine
• Fluoride
• Pesticides
• Plastics
• Pollutants such as dioxins and PCBs
• Solvents
• Toxic metals

While there are many drug therapies out there designed to prevent heart disease, these in themselves can sometimes be toxic. Take the drugs given for high cholesterol, for example. Called statins, these drugs prevent cholesterol from being made. But they also lead to the diminished production of hormones and other substances made from cholesterol.

There is much evidence showing the relationship to inflammation and cardiovascular disease, plaque formation and heart attack. One of the consequences of toxins is they are very proinflammatory. Meaning they cause inflammation. Inflammation has been associated with cancer, heart disease, Alzheimer's and many other health problems.

Avoiding chemicals and detoxifying is a great way not only to control symptoms, but to get to the heart of the matter, no pun intended! Many heart diseases can be controlled by avoiding toxins and following a good nutrition and supplement program.

CHAPTER 16

THE HEALING PROCESS

The Road to Feeling Good Again

"It is my view that you have developed a science all its own. My hope is also that one day you will teach your science to the world. Your endeavors have helped so many people to wellness when they otherwise could not have found a way. In my own life, I would have been gravely ill from severe copper poisoning. I am alive and well because of your help. Targeted Nutritional Analysis is the science of the future.

"I am grateful to have been a part of the development of this science at its early stages and to have worked with you. You are a brilliant scientist disguised as a clinical nutritionist and chiropractor. Blessings to you."

—Alarra

Grand Blanc, Michigan

> *"My legs are less swollen and I used to not want to wear a dress. My liver enzymes are better now, since being on the program. My blood pressure has been better and I'm taking less blood pressure medication now. I couldn't sleep from fungal rash on my back and now it's gone. If I hadn't done this program I wouldn't have believed it. Before I did the program I felt like I was shutting down. I have a better mental attitude. Clearer thinking, more energy, and I'm less stiff upon rising in the morning."*
> —*Jackie*
> *Sarasota, Florida*

Now that you've read this far you know that toxins are all around us. You know they are in your food, in the toiletries you use, in your furniture and rugs, and in the air. They are hard to avoid!

And you also know how toxins affect the body. You know about the toxic body burden, and how the body reacts when it comes into contact with too many toxic chemicals over a period of time. You now understand that a whole host of diseases and disorders, from heart disease to obesity, from autoimmune disorders to neurological problems, have connections to the toxins that we encounter every day.

All of this can seem incredibly overwhelming. After all, chemicals are everywhere! How can we possibly avoid them? The answer is, you can't avoid toxic chemicals entirely. But what you *can* do is make lifestyle and food choices that cut down on your exposure to chemicals. Combine this with a designed detoxification program, plus nutrition and supplements to help your body deal with the toxins it *does* encounter, and your toxic body burden is significantly reduced. And when that happens, you are returned to optimal health!

Avoiding Toxic Chemicals in Daily Life

Here are some lifestyle changes you can make to reduce your daily exposure to chemicals:

- Install "point of entry" filters for your tap and shower water, or an ozone system, or a reverse osmosis system. These will greatly reduce chlorine and other chemicals coming into your home via water.

- If you have a lawn service, ask them not to use pesticides on your lawn. Today, there are many lawn companies that specialize in lawn care without the harmful chemicals.

- Buy certified organic food, and be sure to wash all fruits and veggies before eating them.

- Use the toiletries and household cleaners on our approved list, which appears earlier in this book.

- When you go to the dentist, avoid mercury fillings and don't get the fluoride treatments.

- Use fluoride-free toothpaste

Test Your Toxic Body Burden

Avoiding toxins as you go about your daily life is a great first step. However, what do you do about all those toxins that have already built up in your body over the years? Is there a way to eliminate them?

There is. Actually there are several different tools to evaluate and analyze your toxin burden. Integrative/alternative medicine has been in the forefront of addressing the toxic burden. Laboratory testing, Bioenergetic testing and muscle testing have historically been the three main tools to evaluate your toxic burden.

Dr. Mehmet Oz, the Health Expert on the Oprah Show, has stated these are valid and acceptable tools for better health. A little bit on Dr. Oz's background. He is Professor of Surgery at Columbia University, Director of the Cardiovascular Institute and Complementary Medicine Program at New York Presbyterian Hospital. Dr. Oz is a published author and has been a contributing author to *Newsweek*, *The New England Journal of Medicine* and *Esquire Magazine*.

It is so refreshing to see Medical Doctors embracing Complementary and Alternative medicine. I have been in Complementary Natural Health for over 30 years and "these times they are a changin'!" Changing for the better through more awareness about the importance of nutrition, toxins, detoxification and people actively participating in their own health care.

At Nutrition Wellness Center and the Natural Health Association, (a private membership club) we use a combination of the above mentioned methods in order to evaluate your total toxic burden. Our members are from all over the United States and many of them have us do their nutritional testing from afar. I also have an online internet membership site with many articles and reports I have written which you will have access to with your membership. I will be providing names, addresses and phone numbers of Natural Health Practioners all across the country who provide nutrition, detoxification, and evaluation of your toxic burden.

Here at Nutrition Wellness Center, we have several goals. Our first goal is to raise awareness about the toxins that can potentially destroy our good health.

We don't need to guess what is causing your health problems. Our analysis of your toxic body burden spells it all out for you. Toxic body burden analysis helps eliminate the guesswork and cost of taking supplements or herbs you may *not* need, and specifies your personal nutritional recommendations to give you optimum benefits for the nutritional support you require.

In a day and age when environmental toxins and infectious agents are daily stressors in our lives, these toxins stress our immune, nervous, and hormonal systems. Scientific research supports the relationship between advanced aging and causative factors of many of today's chronic and degenerative diseases. There have also been numerous scientific studies demonstrating the significant benefits that specific nutritional adjuncts have on different body systems by combating environmental toxins and stressors.

The sole purpose of testing for your total toxic body burden is to give individual, specific, and personalized nutritional recommendations to detoxify and support cellular function based on a person's individualized nutritional needs. So you are addressing the *cause*, not merely the *symptoms*. Over the years we found that liver and colon cleanses can be beneficial; but do not address toxins in other tissues such as the brain, thyroid, adrenals, lymphatics, heart and many other areas, thus the evolution of testing for your total toxic body burden and creating a custom wellness program.

So what is involved in our nutritional testing? It's easy! Basically, we mail you a home test kit with instructions for obtaining the urine and saliva samples and how to return them in the mail. We also have a questionnaire you'll mail back to us with your samples. After we receive your paperwork and samples we schedule a time for your report of findings. If you are near southwest Florida, this is done here in our Sarasota office. If you're elsewhere, we schedule your report of findings via telephone. This report is included in the cost of the analysis, and takes about 1-2 hours depending on the complexity of your health issues. The analysis is not a diagnostic test for cancer, heart disease, or any disease process--but rather a comprehensive look into what's *causing* health issues and imbalances. This in-depth analysis enables us to create specific nutritional recommendations and a detoxification program based on your individual needs. Or if you'd prefer to work with a nutritional practitioner in your area, we will be happy to help you find someone.

Detoxification

Once the toxins have been identified, detoxification plans can be formulated. Remember, toxins are one of the main causative factors producing symptoms, sickness, and dis-ease! So what's the key to correction? You guessed it! The elimination of the causative agents, or toxins, from the body and from specific organs and glands.

Depending upon which toxins are determined to be present, specific dietary and detoxification procedures will be put in place. Then and only then can healthy tissue be restored!

After the primary toxins are eliminated, most organs and tissues will heal and repair themselves. At this time any indication from your nutritional evaluation suggesting existing functional/nutritional imbalances are present, would require specific nutritional support for repair and healing. Supplements are used and we eliminate the confusion and guesswork about what you need, what you should take, and for how long.

The maintenance phase includes being retested (as preventative care) to maintain optimal health. This usually requires minimal nutritional support. Due to our daily lifestyles and exposure to environmental stressors, periodic check-ups are recommended.

The time it takes to achieve the above progress is dependent upon the amount of primary toxins, existing lifestyle, present health status, and your follow-through on your individualized program. The time can range from weeks to several months.

As I often say, you can't live in a bubble. And you don't *need to* in order to enjoy good health and freedom from dis-ease. But by minimizing known health risks, and allowing us to help you formulate an individualized plan for wellness, you create a major edge against dis-ease. Take care of yourself ……………... YOU'RE WORTH IT!

- Do you take vitamins or herbal supplements?

- How can you be sure they are the ones YOU NEED?

- Have you asked your doctor about vitamins and supplements?

- Do you rely on sales clerks at your local health food store to know precisely what *your body* needs?

- **Is your doctor highly educated & knowledgeable about the effects of vitamins and supplements or do they just recommend a multi-vitamin for you?**

- Has anyone ever suggested *this product or that product* is good for you? Without any way to find out if it's good for specifically you, how would they know?

- Have you seen ads on TV telling you that YOU NEED their

new multi-vitamin?.... Knowing everyone's body chemistry is a bit different, how can they say that?

- **Is guessing about your own nutritional needs really the right thing to do?**

- Ever wonder how you can find out *specifically* what your body's nutritional needs are?

- Did you know that there is an exciting new way to find out absolutely FREE what your body's own nutritional needs are?

- **What if you could find out all of your own nutritional needs at NO CHARGE to you, would you find out now?**

Want to learn more? Read on.

Over 30 years in the making, I have refined this revolutionary self-help tool to its present precision.

This exciting new analysis takes into account that we all are individuals with individual nutritional needs.

There are many methods to use to assess your nutritional needs that are effective and insightful…blood chemistry tests, saliva & urine analysis all provide helpful information. But frankly not everyone is ready to pay for that type of extensive testing at this very moment. So your best FREE option for your own personalized nutritional assessment is to take this **FREE Nutritional Questionnaire** now.

It has been designed to address stressed organs & systems in the body.

This analysis is one the most comprehensive, highly individualized tools of its kind.

This comprehensive evaluation was originally designed over 30 years ago and since has been reworked, upgraded, expanded, tested and retested to get the best targeted nutritional recommendations from a comprehensive questionnaire.

All recommendations are customized for the individual! No two analyses are the same.

This innovative analysis saves you money by telling you which supplements you DON'T NEED! You'll STOP wasting $$$ on products you may have never needed.

Valued between $100 & $125, this analysis is available to you at <u>NO CHARGE</u>!

Once you've looked over your results, we'll be happy to answer any questions you have....we'll explain anything you may not be knowledgeable about regarding your survey results. Just give us a call. (941)371-1991 or Toll Free (800)222-3610.

"Stop Guessing About <u>Your</u> Targeted Nutritional Recommendations"

Go now to:

www.NewHealthQuiz.com

The New Health Quiz is a nutritional evaluation and <u>NOT</u> a *medical* examination, diagnosis or treatment.

"Why this HEALTH SURVEY can help you resolve Your Health Problems"

Most people think that what causes high blood pressure, chronic pain, allergies, frequent headaches, weight gain and chronic fatigue are the same reasons for everyone.

This is absolutely false. What **causes** specific symptoms in one person could have a totally different **cause** for the same symptoms in another person. I have seen this repeatedly for the last thirty years… same symptoms, different cause. This is why the shotgun approach doesn't work for most people.

I am sure you know someone who has lost weight on a particular weight loss program but it didn't work for *you*. The same is true for all other symptoms. Another good example is allergies, in one person it may be a gut issue, in another person it may be an adrenal issue, or even a liver issue. Addressing the individual **as an individual** produces the best results.

That's why you are taking this individualized HEALTH SURVEY….to pinpoint the organs or glands that are not functioning at their optimum level. Then and only then, do you have a map to address the cause of your specific health issues. Make sense?

I can tell you from my thirty plus years of experience--addressing the "**CAUSE**" versus treating the symptoms has been the only way to resolve health issues, at the same time creating an optimum healthy person.

I have spent years modifying and fine-tuning this survey to improve its accuracy. An imbalance in an organ or system that may show up on your survey may not make sense to you regarding your symptoms. I can assure you--in most cases--it is the organ or systems that need addressing, in order to help resolve your health issues and make you a healthier person as well.

We are happy to discuss any questions you have regarding your survey results…we will explain what you may not be knowledge-able about regarding your survey results.

Go to: **www.NewHealthQuiz.com**

………and find the CAUSE of your symptoms!

Disclaimer
The New Health Quiz is a nutritional evaluation and NOT
a medical examination, diagnosis, or treatment. Taking this
quiz does not imply a doctor-patient relationship.

"Iceberg" - A Model of Dis-ease

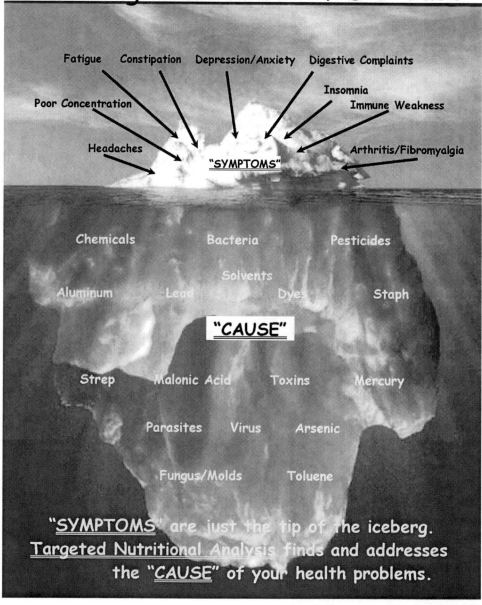

CHAPTER 17

THE 25 DEADLIEST & MOST COMMON TOXINS IN THE USA

Know the Culprits….Knowledge is POWER!

Aluminum

Where It's Hiding . . .

Aluminum is a heavy metal that you can find in some surprising places! Exposure to aluminum comes from food and drink, not from air. Aluminum is commonly found in the leavening agents used in cake mixes, frozen dough, pancake mixes, self-rising flours, and home baking powders. It is also part of the anticaking agent used in table salt, nondairy creamers, and other dry, powdered products. Processed cheese products, particularly the individually wrapped and sliced varieties, often contain aluminum in the emulsifiers to make them smooth. Some foods, such as tea, naturally contain high aluminum levels. Acidic foods, such as fruit juices and coffee, can dissolve aluminum from the cans they are stored in. More important for many people than the intake of foods, however, is the ingestion of aluminum from nonprescription drugs. Buffered aspirin and many antacids contain aluminum. The aluminum content of some antacids ranges from 35 to more than 200 milligrams per dose.

Other sources of aluminum exposure are drinking water, some anti-diarrhea agents and hemorrhoid medications, vaginal douches, antiperspirants, and lipstick. Concentrations tend to be high downwind of such industrial sources as coal-fire power plants, metal smelters, cement manufacturing plants, and waste incinerators. Use of aluminum in the United States amounts to more than five million tons per year.

How It Affects You . . .

Workers exposed to aluminum dust on the job, both in the aluminum fabricating industries and in the production of fireworks, explosives, and alumina abrasives, may develop a lung disease called pulmonary fibrosis. This is a thickening and scarring of the lung tissue around the inhaled particles and can lead to breathlessness similar to emphysema.

The most severe complications have occurred in patients undergoing kidney dialysis.

Aluminum is now suspected, although not proven, to be a factor in the development of Alzheimer's disease. In patients who have died of Alzheimer's, the aluminum content of their brain cells has reached abnormally high concentrations. Experimental animals injected with aluminum also developed the same characteristic symptoms of Alzheimer's patients.

Aluminum may act by interfering with the normal metabolism of nerve cells, rendering them electrically silent and unable to conduct nerve signals.

Aluminum is suspected to cause cardiovascular, neurological, and respiratory issues in people.

Arsenic

Where It's Hiding . . .

Arsenic is used mainly in pesticides and wood preservatives. Most human exposures, about 70% in fact, are to arsenic in food. They are the result of natural occurrence, pesticide residues, and antibiotics given to commercial livestock. Meat, fish, and poultry contain the highest concentrations, and seafood is particularly enriched. Drinking water and air provide relatively smaller exposures, but in the more harmful inorganic form. Cigarette smokers receive an added dose of inorganic arsenic.

Coal burning produces the largest quantity of arsenic waste of any industry because of the large amount of coal burned and the fact that arsenic is a trace contaminant of coal. Studies now show that arsenic is gradually migrating away from such pits and appearing in nearby groundwater.

Did you know? A one-time dose of 60,000 ppb of arsenic will kill you. That's no more than 1/50 the weight of a penny, which shows how dangerous arsenic really is!

Arsenic levels are also high in agricultural areas where arsenic pesticides are used. Arsenic is mixed with other ingredients in wood preservatives, pesticides and drying agents for cotton, glass decolorizers, and other uses. The entire consumption of 20,000 tons per year is imported.

How It Affects You . . .

Lung cancer from inhaling arsenic and skin cancer for swallowing it are the two most dangerous effects of arsenic exposure for the general population.

The Internal Agency for Research on Cancer places inorganic arsenic in its highest classification of cancer-causing substances,

indicating that sufficient evidence exists to judge arsenic as a producer of human concerns.

Other disorders resulting from chronic arsenic exposure are non-cancerous skin lesions, peripheral nerve effects, and cardiovascular changes. Skin disorders include increased pigmentation, wart-like lesions on the palms and soles, and transverse white lines across the nails. Nervous system effects begin with tingling and numbness in the soles and palms, and progress to a widespread and painful neuritis of the upper and lower limbs. Peripheral vascular changes occasionally leading to gangrene have also been reported.

Are Tasteless Toxins on Your Table?

Here are a few facts about pesticides you should know:

- Current law allows 350 pesticides to be used on the food we eat.

- Of the roughly 900 pesticide active ingredients registered in the United States, more than 160 have been classified as known or suspected carcinogens by the United States EPA.

- The highest concentrations of the 13 most toxic pesticides can be found in the following foods (listed in decreasing order of concentrations); tomatoes, beef, potatoes, oranges, lettuce, apples, peaches, pork, wheat, soybeans, beans, carrots, chicken, corn, and grapes.

- Of the 4 billion pounds of pesticides used annually, 1.2 billion pounds are used here in the United States.

- Recent studies have shown 50-70 chemical residues in the fatty tissues of ordinary Americans.

- The highest incidences of cancer, especially leukemia's and lymphomas, occur in people who work on farms. The same is true for Parkinson's disease.

- Over 60,000 registered pesticides are known to damage the nervous system. Most neurological disorders do not develop until 80% of the neurons in a particular area of the brain have been destroyed.

- The Environmental Working Group found at least 66 different illegal pesticides on the 42 fruits and vegetables they tested from local supermarkets. A person eating the USDA's recommended five servings of fruits and vegetables per day will eat illegal pesticides at least 5 times per day.

- Almost 1/4 of all pesticides used in the United States are applied to cotton. Every year half a million tons of cottonseed oil goes into salad dressing, baked goods, and snacks. Another three million tons of cottonseed is fed to beef and dairy cattle.

- In 1997, an Environmental Working Group study found that weed killers came right out of the tap water in 28 of the 29 cities sampled, at levels that routinely exceeded federal standards or health advisories.

- Besides foods, pesticides are also found in plastics, fabrics, mattresses, wallpaper, air fresheners, carpets, paints, toiletries, waxes, leather, and more.

Would you believe that countless numbers of people have told me stories of childhood incidents where they actually *ran behind* pesticide-spraying trucks? DDT, a now banned pesticide, was used in many of our homes while growing up. These tasteless, often odorless toxins have permeated our bodies, our food, our soil, air, and water. We wonder . . . how many neurological diseases and autoimmune disorders have been caused by the slow unseen build-up of pesticides in the brain? How many more Americans will be diagnosed with Parkinson's, Lupus, Rheumatoid Arthritis, Depression, Infertility, Chronic Fatigue, and Birth Defects, and treated with toxic drugs, while the possibility of slow pesticide poisoning stays hidden?

Pesticides are only one environmental toxin that needs to be avoided and removed from the body. When the brain is slowly poisoned from pesticides, the damage can manifest as a dimmer switch works . . . gradually reducing our short-term memory, clarity of thought, reaction time, and many cognitive processes.

People believe that pesticides are only harmful if inhaled or ingested. Well, guess what? The major source of pesticide entry is through the skin. The skin is more susceptible to these toxins than inhalation, as verified by warning labels on pesticide products. Pesticides pose a serious health threat to the adult population, but even more so to our children. Young children are at a primary risk with more skin surface for their size than adults. Young children are playing and breathing toxic residue found in carpeting, indoor/outdoor air, soil, and lawns. Children's hands come in contact with these treated areas and then they are put in their mouths. Pesticide poisoning causes detrimental effects to the underdeveloped nervous system of children.

So why isn't the EPA protecting us against these harmful toxins? The informative book Designer Poisons, by Marion Moses, M.D., gives us evidence that "In 1993, consumers spent 1.2 billion dollars to buy 71 million pounds of home pesticides. The EPA approves pesticides based on efficacy, not safety. Efficacy means pesticides will do what the label says—kill insects, or weeds, or rats, or other pests." Pesticides do to humans what they do to pests. But, in humans it takes much longer to notice the damaging effects.

Aspartame

Where It's Hiding . . .

Aspartame is an artificial sweetener used in all kinds of foods, from diet soda to low-calorie cereal. It is amazing the damage we can do to ourselves in the name of good health!

How It Affects You . . .

Would you believe that complaints about Aspartame account for about 80 percent of the telephone calls received on the FDA food additives hotline?

Despite the lack of evidence regarding toxic effects of aspartame, some scientists are concerned because aspartame contains an amino acid called aspartate that in large doses is known to stimulate the brain excessively. This over-stimulation can damage the brain, perhaps leading to neurological diseases. Studies also indicate that children, especially infants, might be particularly vulnerable to brain damage caused by aspartate-induced over-stimulation of neurons in the brain. Some scientists suggest that pregnant women should avoid ingesting aspartame because infant laboratory animals seem particularly vulnerable to brain damage caused by excessive stimulation to the brain brought about by aspartate.

Benzene

Where It's Hiding . . .

While pumping gasoline, struggling through an organic chemistry class, or cleaning paint brushes, most of us have encountered the compound benzene. Man-made benzene, derived from petroleum and coal, is produced in enormous volume—about 4.6 million tons a year in the United States! Benzene is found in paints, oils, resins, paintbrush cleaners, adhesives, aspirin, deodorants, oven cleaners, asphalt, explosives, pesticides, plastics, detergents, dyes, synthetic rubber, and many other products. As lead is phased out, more benzene is being used.

Because it occurs in so many products, benzene is widely distributed in air and water. It is released into surface water in municipal and industrial wastewater discharges. It is a constituent of emissions from motor vehicles and from major chemical manufacturing and refining industries.

Studies in which people carried personal air quality monitors throughout the course of a normal day revealed that the major source of exposure to benzene is cigarette smoking. Smokers directly breathe the 30 million metric tons of benzene released annually by cigarettes.

How It Affects You . . .

The International Agency for Research on Cancer classifies benzene as a carcinogen. Aplastic anemia, changes in the production of red and white blood cells in the bone marrow, and other effects on the blood are associated with chronic exposure to benzene. Bone marrow changes can occur several years after exposure has ceased. Epidemiological studies link chromosomal aberrations and leukemia to benzene exposure.

Benzene is also a long-term contaminant of groundwater because it can't readily evaporate underground.

Biotoxins

Toxins known as BIOTOXINS are produced by living organisms such as bacteria, fungi and molds. These biotoxins can be more harmful to health than the actual bacteria itself. For example, the organism we know as streptococcus bacteria emits an inflammatory chemical called phenol. It is the phenol that acts as an irritant to tissues. Thus, the pain of a 'strep throat' is actually from the biotoxin called phenol, and not from the strep germ itself.

Most biotoxins are tissue irritants and cause inflammation, often chronically. Scientists know chronic inflammation is associated with many diseases including diabetes, Alzheimer's, heart disease, and even cancer.

When low-level smoldering infections are left unchecked in the body, the cascade of biotoxins can turn an acute infection into a lifelong battle against debilitating health challenges.

Individuals suffering with depression, chronic fatigue syndrome, fibromyalgia, and irritable bowel syndrome (IBS), multiple sclerosis (MS), sick-building syndrome, Bell's palsy, learning disabilities, endometriosis and post-Lyme disease have been helped once the biotoxins were eliminated.

The more stressed the body's pathways of detoxification, the greater the likelihood of biotoxins being present and causing chronic illness.

Chronic Lyme disease is being seen in more areas then ever before in history. Much controversy exists as to what constitutes effective treatment against this disease. New research suggests that a chronic illness may endure long after the lyme pathogens (such as Borrelia burgdorfi and babesia microti) have been killed. Assisting the body's self-cleansing pathways is paramount to ridding the body of biotoxins and restoring good health.

Cadmium

Where It's Hiding . . .

Cadmium is used to galvanize metal parts, as a pigment in paints and plastics, in rechargeable nickel-cadmium batteries, and as a catalyst and preservative in the plastics industry. Ceramic glazes, oil paints, and other art supplies often contain cadmium-based pigments.

Most important sources of cadmium contamination are the burning of fossil fuels, municipal and medical waste, and sewage sludge. Cadmium and zinc mining, metal processing, electroplating, plastics and dye manufacturing, the manufacture and disposal of nickel-cadmium batteries, municipal wastewater treatment, and application of phosphate fertilizers are all sources of cadmium in soil, water, and other sediments.

Cadmium is a trace contaminant in fertilizers and is slowly but steadily building up in agricultural soils. This may become the most important source of cadmium in the future. Currently, food contributes 80 to 90 percent of the cadmium dose received by most people. Flounder, mussels, scallops, oysters, and crab usually contain the highest concentrations of cadmium among marine species. Smoking is another significant source of exposure.

How It Affects You . . .

Inhaled cadmium is associated with lung cancer in people. The EPA classified it as a probable human carcinogen. Although cadmium induced lung cancer has been formally linked only to the heavy concentrations normally associated with occupational exposure to cadmium fumes, chronic exposure to low levels of cadmium may also result in progressive lung diseases such as emphysema and chronic bronchitis. Chronic exposure to cadmium is also associated with a wide range of other diseases, including heart disease, anemia, skeletal weakening, depressed immune system response, and kidney and liver disease. Kidney function is not affected until cadmium concentration reaches a critical level. Then, signs of kidney dysfunction become apparent. At this time, the excretion of cadmium increases dramatically but, unfortunately, kidney damage is irreversible. High levels of cadmium in the body are associated with brittle bones. Cadmium-caused combination of brittle bones and kidney damage is called itai-itai disease. High concentrations of cadmium in the air can cause chest pain, coughing, and lung problems as well as chills, muscle aches, nausea, vomiting, and diarrhea four to 10 hours following exposure.

Chlorine

Where It's Hiding . . .

It's true that toxins and pathogens found in water have been known to cause many diseases. But did you know that what is put in your water can also make you sick? That's right. In an attempt to purify water, chlorine is added.

About two thirds of our exposure to chlorine is due to inhalation of steam, as well as skin absorption, when showering and bathing.

How It Affects You . . .

The French, with their lower cancer rates, have made red wine famous for its health benefits. But there is another side to their low cancer rates that most people don't know. And here it is: the French do not drink chlorinated water. Instead, they ozonate their water to purify it.

According to the U.S. Council of Environmental Quality, "Cancer risk among people drinking chlorinated water is 93% higher than among those whose water does not contain chlorine.

It may cause heart disease, too. In a study headed up by Dr. Joseph Price, author of *Coronaries/Cholesterol/Chlorine*, chickens were used as test subjects. Two groups of several hundred birds were observed throughout their life spans. One group was given water with chlorine, and the other group was given water without chlorine. The group raised with chlorine, when autopsied, showed some level of circulatory disease in every specimen, while the group without chlorine had no incidence of disease. The group without chlorine also grew faster, larger, and displayed better health.

Chlorine may also cause breast cancer, bladder cancer, and senility. Chlorine, simply put, is a pesticide! And as such, it does what it is supposed to do. As we continue to ingest and absorb chlorine, it destroys the cells and tissues in our bodies.

Chromium

Where It's Hiding . . .

Chromium is one of our biggest air pollutants. It is used in metal finishing, chromium chemicals production, chromium pigments for paints and textiles, leather tanning, and some wood preservatives. It is also in electrical power plant cooling towers to prevent corrosion in the cooling loops. Total consumption of chromium in the United States is approximately 500,000 tons per year, of which 60% goes to metallurgical uses, 21% to chemicals production, and 18% for use in lining furnaces.

How It Affects You . . .

Chromium can produce liver and kidney damage, internal hemorrhage, dermatitis, respiratory damage, and lung cancer, although dramatic cases of chromium poisoning are rarely seen today because of improvements in industrial safety and hygiene. Longer-term exposures to the respiratory tract and skin can produce perforated and ulcerated nasal septa, inflammation of the nasal passages, frequent nose bleeds, and skin ulcers. These effects are usually seen after industrial exposure.

Where are you most likely to run into chromium? Well, what if I told you it was commonly used in leather, cement, brewers yeast, wood preservatives, priming paint, glue, and paint pigment. All fairly common things, right? If you get an allergic reaction on your skin after handling any of these things, chances are you are reacting to the chromium

And here's something else. **The EPA rates chromium among the top one-fourth of substances ranked for carcinogenic potency.** Workers in the chromium chemicals industry in the United States, Great Britain, West Germany, and Japan show a clear association between chromium exposure and lung cancer. Lab experiments further confirm that chromium compounds can damage genetic material. Other studies on laboratory animals show that this form of chromium can cause fetal malformations and reproductive problems.

Electromagnetic Fields & Radiation

The spectrum of electromagnetism includes x-rays, radon gas, microwaves, radio, TV, telephone, cell phones, electrical power, ultraviolet, ELF (extra low frequency waves) and more frequencies.

Radon—a Silent Killer in Your Home?

Radon, for example, poses a serious threat in millions of American homes. Radon is a radioactive by-product of uranium decay, seeping up through the ground in the form of a gas. The NCI (the National Cancer Institute) states that radon may be responsible for at least 30,000 lung cancer deaths each year, second only to tobacco as a lung cancer cause. The most tightly insulated homes tend to concentrate radon gas inside the house more than homes whose doors and windows allow for air flow. Radon monitors are available at many home improvement and hardware stores.

The parts of the U.S. most affected by radon are:

Parts of NY State

Northwest New Jersey

Eastern Pennsylvania

Appalachian mountain area

Parts of Montana, South Dakota, Colorado & Florida

Microwave Oven Dangers

The dangers of microwave ovens are often ignored in the United States, but they are well-known to the Russians. For many years in Russia microwaves were banned entirely. Some of the findings by Russian scientists include:

- Microwaved foods lose 60 to 90% of the vital energy field and microwaving accelerates the structural disintegration of foods.

- Microwaving creates cancer-causing agents within milk and cereals.

- Microwaving alters elemental food-substances, causing digestive disorders.

- Microwaving alters food chemistry, which can lead to malfunctions in the lymphatic system and degeneration of the body's ability to protect itself against cancerous growths.

- Microwaved foods lead to a higher percentage of cancerous cells in the bloodstream.

- Microwaving altered the breakdown of elemental substances when raw, cooked, or frozen vegetables were exposed for even a very short time and free radicals were formed.

- Microwaved foods caused stomach and intestinal cancerous growths, a general degeneration of peripheral cellular tissues, and a gradual breakdown of the digestive and excretive systems in a statistically high percentage of people.

- Microwaved foods lowered the body's ability to utilize B-complex vitamins, Vitamin C, Vitamin E, essential minerals and lipotrophics.

- Another study in Vienna, Austria warned that microwaving breast milk "can lead to structural, functional and immunological changes," and that microwaves transform the amino acid L-proline into D-proline, a proven toxin to the nervous system, liver and kidneys.

Are X-Rays Dangerous?

X-rays, a.k.a. ionizing radiation, cause disruption of the molecule, causing it to be electrically unbalanced. The DNA of the cells is damaged, potentially leading to cancer. Diagnostic x-rays (radiographs) are sometimes necessary; but taking anti-oxidants regularly helps protect against cellular damage. The risks versus benefits of medical and dental radiation must be seriously weighed before submitting to any such procedures. This would include dental x-rays, mammograms, spinal/joint x-rays, nuclear medicine studies, radioactive implanted seeds, and radiation oncology therapies.

What If I live Near a Power Plant?

Of 35 international studies on electromagnetic radiation, 33 made a conclusive link with cancers. There was also a 300% increase in brain tumors in children whose mothers used electric blankets during pregnancy.

Exposure to EMF (electromagnetic fields) is most dangerous when in close proximity. Many electrical and electronic devices cause muscle weakness.

These include:

Motors

Transformers

Fluorescent lights

Battery powered & digital watches & clocks

Electric blankets, waterbed heaters

Video display terminals (TV's, computer screens, video games)

Another example of how EMF affects the human body—an ionizing smoke detector within 60 feet of the bed can diminish the male and female sex drive. Both the heart and the nervous system are electrical and susceptible to other types of electrical currents.

Because you have billions of electrons in your body, any magnetic field *near* the body (a motor, an electrical appliance, etc) causes your electrons to move just as they do inside a wire. This is how cell phones cause changes in brain function, by moving electrons in an abnormal flow pattern.

Cell Phones and Brain Cancer Linked

Brain cancer has surpassed leukemia as the number one cancer killer in children. Australia has seen an increase in pediatric brain cancer of 21% in just one decade. In Europe and the United Kingdom, a 40% brain tumor increase in the last 20 years has been reported.

Although cell phone radiation is of low intensity, it is the oscillatory similarity between this pulsed microwave radiation and certain electrochemical activities within your body that raises serious concerns, according to the study *"Physics and biology of mobile telephony,"* published in *The Lancet,* medical journal.

Your body is essentially a very sensitive electromagnetic instrument, controlled by highly complex and orderly oscillatory electrical processes. The pulsating low-intensity microwaves from mobile phones can exert subtle, non-thermal influences on human biology, simply because microwaves are *waves.* Therefore, much in the same way as a radio can receive interference; your biological processes can be interfered with by the incoming oscillatory aspect of incoming radiation.

Highly organized electrical processes at the cellular level are especially vulnerable to interference from cell phone radiation, because their frequency happens to fall within the microwave range.

To minimize exposure and risk:

- Prohibit the use of cell phones by children unless in an emergency (they are more vulnerable then adults, because of smaller skulls & developing brains)

- Reduce cell phone use as much as possible

- Use a land line phone instead of a cell phone as much as possible

- If you must use a portable home phone—use an older model that operates at a 900MHz frequency (they do not broadcast constantly when no call is being made)

- Turn off your cell phone when not in use

- Keep cell phones at least 6 inches away from your body when not in use

- Use headset technology (shielded wire & air-tube headsets avoid wires going directly to the head)

Fluoride

Where It's Hiding . . .

Fluoride is a synthetic chemical that belongs to the halogen family. It is most often used for the prevention of cavities in products like toothpaste, mouthwash, and in treatments that you get at your dentist.

Fluoride can also be found in many city water systems. Like chlorine, it is added because of supposed health benefits. You can even buy bottled water now with added fluoride. People who have well water or water that does not have fluoride treatment are often given fluoride drops to administer to their children when they are young and growing, in order to prevent tooth decay.

How It Affects You . . .

But if fluoride is so good for you, why has it been labeled a suspected carcinogen? And why has it been banned in many European countries?

Fluoride has been shown to cause thyroid disease. Furthermore, despite its widespread use in the dental industry, studies have shown that it doesn't reduce cavities after all. In fact, it may even cause dental deformity and bone disease.

The Greater Boston Physicians for Social Responsibility found that fluoride interferes with brain function, and can cause a lowered IQ in children. It has also been shown to cause bone cancer in rats.

Dr. Cornelius Steelink, Emeritus Professor of the Department of Chemistry at the University of Arizona in Tucson, AZ studied fluoride exposure in 26,000 school children. The results showed the more fluoride a child drank the more cavities the child experienced. **The U.S. Environmental Protection Agency has classified fluoride as *more toxic than lead but less toxic than arsenic.***

Food Colors

Where They're Hiding . . .

We come into contact with food dyes and colors every single day. As a matter of fact, it's hard to eat a meal these days without ingesting synthetic chemicals. Food dyes are even used in products that you wouldn't suspect, like toothpaste!

The fact is, the American food industry puts over 3,000 tons of food color into processed foods every year. Wow! And here's another little-known fact: synthetic food colors are made from molecules derived from petroleum or coal tar. Now, are these things that you really want on your plate?

If you are wondering where food dyes are most commonly used, you can find them in soda, candy, dessert mixes, commercially prepared baked goods, sausages and hot dogs, toothpaste, and cosmetics. Red No. 40 and Yellow No. 5 and No. 6 make up more than 90% of the food dyes used in the United States. Using data provided by the FDA, one consumer group calculated that some children consume as much as three pounds of food dye by their twelfth birthdays.

How It Affects You . . .

The question isn't really whether food dyes cause cancer. That has been proven in lab test after lab test using mice, rats, rabbits, and even monkeys. Rather, the question is how high a dose a human needs to eat before becoming affected. Here are some of the health affects associated with food dyes:

- Red No. 3—thyroid tumors, chromosomal damage

- Red No. 40—lymphatic tumors

- Blue No. 1—chromosomal damage

- Blue No. 2—brain tumors

- Green No. 3—bladder tumors

- Yellow No. 5—thyroid and lymphatic tumors, allergy

- Yellow No. 6—kidney tumors, chromosomal damage, allergy

Another toxic chemical that has been found in food dyes is **lanthanides**. These are rare earth metals that have a magnetic quality second only to iron. They fill your cells with iron and calcium deposits, and disturb your body's own DNA production, causing cellular mutation.

Lanthanides are most often found in fruit and veggie dyes. So even the food you think is healthy may not be! In fact, lanthanides have a disabling effect on the immune system. See, normally the body digests unhealthy cells. But cells choked with iron and calcium are not able to hoist a "flag" that tells your body to digest them. So lanthanides prevent self digestion, which is the very mechanism that causes tumors to dissolve.

Where else can you find lanthanides? Well, in addition to fruits and vegetables, you can find lanthanides in pesticides, as well as in dental fillings.

Formaldehyde

Where It's Hiding . . .

What if I told you that you most likely come into contact with formaldehyde each and every day? That's right. Because if it's widespread distribution, virtually the entire population is exposed to formaldehyde.

In 1985, more than 5.7 billion pounds of formaldehyde were produced for an enormous variety of purposes. The chemical is used to make a diverse selection of consumer products such as molded plastic telephones, dinnerware, particleboard, plywood, foam mattresses, insulation, cosmetics, and drugs. It is used as a preservative, an embalming fluid, a fumigant, and a disinfectant. It is also a normal combustion product found in cigarette smoke, wood smoke, automobile exhaust, and emissions from incinerators and power plants.

Formaldehyde is in many of the vaccines we give our children, the permanent press fabrics we wear, and in the furniture we relax in. As a matter of fact, I can guarantee that the room you are sitting in right now as you read this has furnishings made with formaldehyde. Both plywood and particle board are typically used in subflooring, countertops, cabinets, paneling, and furniture, and more than 90% of furniture made and sold in the United States is built with pressed wood products.

How It Affects You . . .

The EPA has concluded, after much debate with the Formaldehyde Institute, that formaldehyde is a probably human carcinogenic. The epidemiological studies suggest an increased incidence in brain tumors, leukemia, and cirrhosis of the liver among professional workers. Laboratory studies indicate that formaldehyde causes nasal cancer in rats and that it appears to cause mutations in bacteria, yeasts, Drosophila, and mammalian and human cells.

Signs of poisoning can included abdominal pain, anxiety, irritation of the nose and throat, depression of the central nervous system, coma, convulsions, diarrhea, headache, nausea, vomiting, and various respiratory problems such as bronchitis, pneumonia, or pulmonary edema. Lower levels of exposure can cause dermatitis, cough, and decreased lung capacity. Classic symptoms of low-level formaldehyde exposure include runny nose, sore throat, sleeping difficulties, sinus irritation, chest pain, frequent nausea, and bronchitis.

Lead

Where It's Hiding . . .

We all know about the effects of lead, a common industrial metal, on children. After all, the campaign against lead paint has been widespread in the United States. As a result of that campaign, most of us are aware that thousands of preschool children who have inadvertently eaten chips and flakes of lead dust from old buildings, have been poisoned and suffered irreversible brain damage.

But what you need to know is that lead isn't just found in the paint of old buildings. Lead is in our air, our soil, our water, and our food. As a matter of fact, food accounts for more than 60% of blood levels, air inhalation accounts for approximately 30%, and water for 10%. Why is there lead in our food? Well, lead gets into our food by crops absorbing it from the soil, dry fallout from the air onto leaves, absorption from cooking water, contamination during processing, solder from cans, and leaching from storage material.

How It Affects You . . .

Lead causes severe health problems, at relatively low levels in the body. It affects the human nervous system, the production of blood cells, kidneys, reproductive system, and behavior. The symptoms can be vague and hard to pin down, but common symptoms of lead poisoning include pallor, vomiting, abdominal pain, constipation, listlessness, stupor, loss of appetite, irritability, and loss of muscular coordination.

Malonic Acid

Where It's Hiding . . .

Malonic acid is a chemical substance which occurs naturally in some plant foods and unnaturally in processed food, medicines, heated oils, and the plastic of dental restorations. Malonic acid is also made by some parasites and living organisms.

Malonic acid is not natural for humans! In fact, nothing in scientific literature indicates that it is a metabolite.

There's a good reason why we don't have free malonic acid in our bodies anywhere. It is an extremely potent metabolic inhibitor. In whatever organ it is found, your metabolism slows down. As a matter of fact, it almost grinds to a halt! What's the end result? The organ can't use as much oxygen, nor can it make as much energy as it should. Consequently, we make fewer amino acids and less protein. And what does this lead to? Lowered immunity.

Malonic acid can be found in all kinds of healthy foods, from alfalfa sprouts to wheat grass. So should you avoid these foods? Well, not entirely. These foods are nutritious and have wonderful properties. A little later, we'll talk about how to detoxify your system. Until your detoxification is complete, foods with malonic acid, as well as all fried foods and heated oils, should be avoided.

Foods Containing Malonic Acid

• alfalfa sprouts • apricots • araica • black beans • great northern beans • lima beans • mung beans • navy beans • red kidney beans • black olives • broccoli • butternut squash • carrots • chaparral • chocolate • ginger root skin • grape jam • green zucchini • seaweed • limes • mangos • nori seaweed • purple onions • oranges • papaya • parsnips • passion fruit • persimmons • radish • red skin of peanuts • tamari soy sauce • tomatoes • turnips • rutabaga • wheat grass

How It Can Affect You . . .

Malonic acid is known for causing a host of ill effects, including lowering the immune system, causing oxygen to be cut off from organs, kidney toxicity, raising cholesterol, reducing the ability to fight infection, increasing the formation of fatty acids, slowing, or even stopping, metabolism, causing tumors, and fluid retention and swelling.

Mercury

Where It's Hiding . . .

Anyone who turns on the evening news now knows that we are all at risk of mercury poisoning. It is unfortunate that many types of fish, long considered to have health benefits and to be an important part of the diet, are now off limits due to mercury contamination.

That's right. While liquid mercury and mercury vapor continue to be threats, methyl mercury in fish and fish products is by far the largest source of mercury exposure at 94%.

According to the EPA, those who eat more than 30 pounds of fish a year are in the high-risk group. Freshwater fish tend to have slightly higher levels than marine species.

Mercury in fish is what we most often hear about. But you can also find mercury in the manufacture of electrical equipment, batteries, mercury cells in smoke detectors, and mercury lamps and switches. It can also be found in the production of chlorine and caustic soda, as an antimildew agent in paints, in industrial and control instruments, and in other products.

How It Can Affect You . . .

Mercury is a potential neurotoxin, capable of causing severe brain damage in developing fetuses and mild tremors and emotional disturbances in exposed adults. Mercury has been responsible for numerous poisonings in the past.

Mild exposure can cause memory loss, tremors, emotional instability, insomnia, and loss of appetite. Introversion appears to be the most prominent personality trait in affected people. At moderate exposures, more significant mental disorders and motor disturbances, as well as kidney damage, are seen. More severe cases show constriction of vision, diminished hearing, speech disorders, shaky movements, and unsteady gaits.

Methylene Chloride

Where It's Hiding . . .

Innocent acts such as using hairspray and enjoying a cup of decaf can expose you to methylene chloride. Methylene chloride is also the most common chemical used to remove paint. In addition to being found in aerosols and decaffeinated beverages, methylene chloride is used as an ingredient in fumigants, pesticides, and industrial cleaning solutions, as well as in shoe polish, fabric waterproofing, fire extinguishers, air deodorizers, and spot removers.

About 80% of methylene chloride produced each year is released into the atmosphere immediately following its use. Considering that domestic production is estimated at 300,000 tons annually, there's quite a bit of this toxic chemical in the air!

How It Can Affect You . . .

The way methylene chloride affects the body is complicated, as it decomposes into carbon monoxide in the body. So whatever toxic effects you may feel are most likely caused by the carbon monoxide, and not by the chemical itself. Warning signs of overexposure include headache, fatigue, giddiness, irritability, and numbness in the extremities. Damage to the liver and central nervous system is also possible as a result of chronic exposure to the solvent. Heart arrhythmias and death have been ascribed to excessively high levels of solvent in the air.

Methylene chloride may cause cancer. National Toxicology Program inhalation bioassay tests found clear evidence of carcinogenicity. As a matter of fact, the EPA classifies methylene chloride as a probable human carcinogen.

Another thing that is important for you to know: absorbed methylene chloride is distributed through the body and easily crosses the blood-brain barrier and the placenta. It can also be found in the breast milk of exposed women.

MSG

Where It's Hiding…..

"MSG (monosodium glutamate) is a flavoring agent which used to be in baby food to please the parent's taste. It is used in salad dressings, canned soups, processed cheeses, frozen pizza, beer, broths, Chinese food, dry roasted nuts, soup mixes, vegetables (packed with sauce), canned meats, croutons, tomato sauces, bouillon cubes, bread crumbs, meat tenderizers, frozen spinach packages, seafood (packaged), tomato pastes and frankfurters."

MSG in various forms is found in foods such as Campbell's soups, some flavors of Doritos, Lay's flavored potato chips, Betty Crocker Hamburger Helper, Heinz canned gravy, Swanson frozen prepared meals and Kraft salad dressings.

Popular restaurants enhance the tastes of many of their menu items using MSG. Burger King, McDonald's, Wendy's, Taco Bell, TGIF, Chili's, Applebee's, Denny's, and KFC are among the establishments using MSG liberally.

Hidden MSG

MSG may not be labeled as MSG, it's also called:

Monosodium Glutamate
Hydrolyzed Vegetable Protein
Hydrolyzed Protein
Hydrolyzed Plant Protein
Plant Protein Extract
Sodium Caseinate
Calcium Caseinate
Yeast Extract
Textured Protein (including TVP)
Autolyzed Yeast
Hydrolyzed Oat Flour
Corn Oil

So what good is MSG? According to John Erb, in <u>The Slow Poisoning of America,</u> MSG is added to food for the addictive effect it has on the human body. The MSG manufacturers themselves admit that it addicts people to their product. It makes people choose their product over others, and makes people eat more of it than they would if MSG wasn't added. It has been called "nicotine for food" and no maximum limit has been set by the FDA on how much MSG can be added to food.

How It Affects You…..

MSG triples the amount of insulin the pancreas creates, causing rats and most likely humans to become obese. Scientists create morbidly obese rats by injecting them with MSG, then using them as test subjects for diet and diabetes drug studies.

More studies cited in <u>The Slow Poisoning of America</u> show the link between MSG and diabetes, MSG and migraines and other headaches, MSG and autism, MSG and ADHD, even MSG and Alzheimer's.

There is also evidence that MSG "could possibly aggravate or even precipitate many of today's epidemic neurodegenerative brain diseases such as Parkinson's disease, Huntington's disease, ALS, and Alzheimer's disease." He asks, "Would you be concerned if you knew that these excitotoxin food additives are a particular risk if you have diabetes, or have ever had a stroke, brain injury, brain tumor, seizure, or have suffered from hypertension, meningitis or viral encephalitis?"

As food manufacturers continue to put profits ahead of our health, we must be on guard against sources of hidden MSG in foods and beverages and strive to avoid them.

Mycotoxins

Mycotoxins are often overlooked as a causative factor in disease and illness. A mycotoxin is a chemical produced by a yeast, mold or fungus. These mycotoxins suppress the immune system and cause inflammation.

When foods are stored or transported in darkness or dampness, or for extended periods of time, the potential for mold, yeast and fungal growth increases. Wherever yeast, mold and fungus are--there are mycotoxins being made in the same place.

The FDA stated, "Mycotoxins are considered unavoidable contaminants in foods and feeds because agronomic (farming) technology has not yet advanced to the stage at which preharvest infection of susceptible crops by fungi can be eliminated."

Several mycotoxins are cancer-causing. One of them is called AFLATOXIN. The FDA adds, "The alflatoxins have received greater attention than any of the other mycotoxins because of their demonstrated carcinogenic effects in susceptible animals and their acute toxic effects in humans."

Where It's Hiding…..

Primarily made by a fungus called aspergillus, aflatoxin is often present in bread, beans, nuts, beer, wine, apple cider vinegar, syrups, potato peels, cereals, orange juice, pasta, animal feed and cow's milk.

How It Affects You….

It's destructive to the liver, reduces oxygen to the brain, and it usually is found at tumor sites. Tumor formation from alflatoxin was caused in ducklings, ferrets, rats, and trout in animal studies in the 1960's. The carcinogenic effects of aflatoxin mainly affect the kidneys, intestines, stomach and trachea.

Another mycotoxin, ZEARALANONE, is a danger to good health.

Where It's Hiding…..

From fusarium mold, this mycotoxin hides in corn, corn meal, corn chips, popcorn, brown rice and other foods.

How It Affects You…..

Acting as an estrogen-like chemical, zearalenone is capable of causing PMS, ovarian cysts, prostate hyperplasia, pre-puberty sexual development in children, and obesity, especially in cattle. It can cause the thymus gland to atrophy and lowers immune response. It also blocks detoxification of benzene from the cells.

GLIOTOXIN is a mycotoxin which also can be very damaging yet often goes undetected.

Where It's Hiding…..

Growing on grains, nuts, sugar cane, sorghum and more, species of candida albicans, trichoderma, penicillum and aspergillus all emit gliotoxin.

How It Affects You…..

This mycotoxin may make candida albicans infections harder to combat. It also causes DNA breakage in spleen cells. It leads to cell death of lymph cells, liver cells, thymus cells, and bone marrow cells. It has been associated with MS, possibly leading to the neuropathological feature of MS, such as the blood-brain barrier involvement and demyclination. Gliotoxin also induces free radical damage.

Other mycotoxins such as 3-NITROPROPRIONIC ACID (3-NP) can cause seizures and convulsions. OCHRATOXIN, found in bread, beans, grapes, milk, flour, and cocoa beans is highly toxic to kidney cells. It can also lead to iron-deficiency anemia. In a study in Germany, 56% of human blood samples were positive for ochratoxin. A mycotoxin called T-2 toxin can lead to high blood pressure and kidney disease. ERGOT, found in alcoholic beverages, is a liver-poisoning mycotoxin which is believed to be a factor in alcoholism. It may be the cause of the "Jekyll and Hyde" behavior seen in some alcoholics.

Many other mycotoxins exist in our foods that are present in nuts, seeds, grains, grain-fed cattle and from other sources. They are all suppressive to the immune system and cause inflammation. Although cooking can destroy many molds and fungi, high temperatures *do not* destroy mycotoxins.

Nickel

Where It's Hiding . . .

You may expect that industrial workers such as nickel refining and fabricating workers, stainless steel makers, welders, electroplaters, battery makers, jewelers, spray painters, paint makers, and varnish workers are exposed to nickel. But did you also know that beauticians are highly exposed because of the nickel content in shampoos and hair sprays?

Nickel also can be found in tobacco smoke. That kind of nickel, nickel carbonyl, may be the most hazardous type of nickel.

How It Can Affect You . . .

Cancers of the lung, nasal passages, and possibly the larynx are the most serious effects of nickel exposure, but these are probably limited to occupational exposures. Nickel-plating workers and welders exposed to various nickel compounds have developed allergic lung reactions such as asthma, loss of the sense of smell, and severe nasal injuries.

Animal studies have provided compelling evidence that nickel causes cancer. The EPA has concluded that nickel subsulfide causes cancer in humans.

Nickel contact dermatitis, a form of skin eczema or rash, is the most common health effect among the general public. The fact that nickel compounds produce cancer, however, indicates their potential to affect genetic material.

PCBs and PBBs

Where They're Hiding . . .

Four decades after their introduction to the world market, the organochlroine compounds called PCBs were linked to extensive global contamination and serious human illness. By the late 1960s, significant levels of PCBs were being detected in the air, soil, water, sediments, fish, and other wildlife, not to mention human tissues throughout the world.

Where can you find PCBs? PCBs have been used extensively for insulating and cooling electrical equipment, such as transformers and capacitors, and in hydraulic fluids and lubricants. In such applications, the flow of PCBs to the environment is restricted.

So why are there so many PCBs in our environment, and how did they get there? Widespread environmental distribution of PCBs is a result of their use in plasticizers, inks and dyes, as part of pesticide preparation, in adhesives, as protective surfacc coatings for wood, and in carbonless copy paper.

How It Can Affect You . . .

Are PCBs toxic? You bet! Symptoms associated with PCB poisoning include chloracne, increased pigmentation of the fingernails and gums, changes in the immune system, and respiratory distress.

Furthermore, laboratory studies show that PCBs produce a variety of unwanted effects in diverse test animals. PCBs can cross the placenta and are toxic to the embryo, causing numerous adverse reproductive effects, particularly increased stillbirths, spontaneous abortions, and fetal absorptions.

PCBs are classified as human carcinogens. Rodent tests indicate that PCBs cause liver cancer and possibly stomach cancer. Also, an unexplained association exists between high PCB levels in the blood and both elevated cholesterol levels and elevated blood pressure.

Perchlorate

Where It's Hiding . . .

New scientific evidence clearly shows that perchlorate is a much greater public health threat than previously realized. Tests of almost 3,000 human urine and breast milk samples, long with tests of more than 1,000 fruits, vegetables, cow's milk, beer, and wine samples, reveal that perchlorate exposure in the population is pervasive.

The vast majority of perchlorate manufactured in the United States is used by the Department of Defense to make solid rocket and missile fuel, while smaller amounts of perchlorate are also used to make firework and road flares. According to the Environmental Working Group's latest data, perchlorate is known to be contaminating at least 160 public drinking water systems in 26 states.

Perchlorate has been found in a wide variety of domestic and imported produce, with some of the highest levels being found in oranges, grapes, raspberries, apricots, melons, lettuce, tomatoes, basil, kale, spinach, and asparagus, among others.

How It Can Affect You . . .

With the amount of perchlorate being found in the nation's food and drinking water, it should come as no surprise that it is showing up in people's bodies as well. Perchlorate acts by inhibiting the thyroid's ability to take up the nutrient iodine, which is a key building block for thyroid hormones. If the thyroid gland does not have enough iodide for a sufficient period of time, the body's thyroid hormone levels will eventually drop. This is called hypothyroidism, which causes fatigue, depression, anxiety, unexplained weight gain, hair loss, and low libido. More serious, however, are the effects of thyroid disruption in the developing fetus and child; small changes in maternal thyroid levels during pregnancy have been associated with reduced IQs in children. Fetuses, infants, and children who experience more significant changes in hormone levels may suffer mental retardation, loss of hearing or speech, abnormal testicular development, or deficits in motor skills.

Styrene

Where It's Hiding . . .

How often do you encounter and handle something made with plastic during the day? Everyday things like your automobile tires and the pipes your plumbing runs through, from the ink in your printer to the plastic wrap around your sandwich, contains a toxic chemical called styrene.

Today, styrene is one of the most widely used chemicals in the United States, particularly in consumer products. To get an idea of styrene's widespread use, consider that it is used in the following products: automobile tires, PVC pipe, adhesives, photographic film, copy paper, toner, ink, auto parts, plastic food wrap, Styrofoam cups and trays, combs, cushions, eyeglass lenses, bottles, boxes, jars, and kitchen utensils.

Food and water stored in refrigerators with plastic interiors can contain styrene, as can commercial hickory wood smoke flavor and cigarette smoke.

How It Can Affect You . . .

So how does styrene get inside of you? Well, it can be absorbed through the skin, respiratory system, and gastrointestinal tract. Styrene is associated with suppressed estrogen production in females and high-frequency hearing loss.

Teflon: A sticky situation about non-stick surfaces

This modern day toxin is found in Teflon cookware, Silverstone cookware, Stainmaster carpet, Gore-Tex water-resistant clothing and grease-resistant coatings for food packaging. (grease-resistant pizza boxes, fast food containers, microwave popcorn bags, packaging for bakery items, drinks and candy)

The family of Teflon coating chemicals was discovered in 1938 by a DuPont scientist and introduced as a commercial product in 1946. Teflon-related products have been in the market place for over 40 years with estimated sales at 2 billion dollars per year. Believing this new non-stick surface would make our lives easier; millions of Americans began using non-stick cookware on a daily basis.

Why the concern about Teflon now? Recent findings show that 95% of Americans have detectable levels of Teflon-related chemicals in their blood. Toxicity occurs when the non-stick materials are overheated. Polymer fume fever is the term when individuals are sickened by toxic Teflon emissions. Symptoms include chest tightness, malaise, shortness of breath, headache, chills, cough, sore throat and fever.

Perflurooctanic acid, (PFOA) the chemical used to make Teflon, causes cancer, birth defects, and other health problems in animals. Even DuPont admits Teflon will kill birds when heated to moderately high temperatures.

These PFOA's are persistent and do not break down. Research at John Hopkins Hospital has found PFOA in the umbilical cord blood of 99% of newborns tested over a 5 month period.

The Environmental Working Group looked at 16 peer-reviewed studies detailing 50 years worth of experiments showing that Teflon decomposes into 15 types of toxic gases and particles.

Teflon exposure has been linked to death of immune cells, liver damage, high cholesterol levels in children, obesity, thyroid dysfunction, and prostate damage. After hiding data showing the harmful effects of Teflon for 16 years, DuPont has now been forced to re-formulate these chemicals. The sad part is that their replacement chemicals have had no public assessments, and may in fact, be more harmful than the original chemicals.

Toluene

Where It's Hiding . . .

As long as there are cars, trucks, and other petroleum burning engines around us, then we'll have to contend with toluene.

Toluene is a gasoline additive, but is also used as a strong solvent for model glues, paints, inks, resins, and adhesives. It is also used to manufacture detergents, dyes, lacquers, linoleum, perfumes, pharmaceuticals, saccharin, and TNT.

The United States produces about three million tons of toluene each year, much of which ends up in the air through vapors from cars, trucks, and plane exhaust. Cigarette smoking is another form of toluene.

How It Can Affect You . . .

Toluene vapors aggravate the respiratory tract, depress the central nervous system, and damage the liver and kidneys. The early symptoms of toluene exposure can include some combination of the following: fatigue, weakness, confusion, euphoria, dizziness, headaches, dilated pupils, insomnia, extreme light sensitivity, and skin irritation.

Xylene

Where It's Hiding . . .

Look around your home. If you are like most people, chances are you have things like paint, paint remover, nail polish, air fresheners, degreasing cleaners, lacquers, glues, and marking pens lying around.

Well, you should know that these items contain xylene, a chemical used by the petrochemical industry to make other chemicals including solvents, plastics, and pharmaceuticals. More than 6,000 tons of the chemical are released into the air each year during industrial processing!

Xylene is a hydrocarbon, just like benzene and toluene. However, among the three, it is the most toxic.

How It Can Affect You . . .

High concentrations of xylene in the air can cause irritation to the eyes and nose, coughing, hoarseness, and even pulmonary edema. Continued inhalation at levels that cause irritation leads to symptoms that resemble drunkenness, including slowed reaction time, poor balance, and central nervous system depression or agitation, followed by unconsciousness, tremors, and restlessness.

++

Get the latest information on NUTRITION & TOXICITY from:

www.HowToxicAreYou.com/blog

MEET THE WRITER

James H. Martin, N.M.D., D.C.C.N., D.A.C.B.N.,F.A.A.I.M.,is an established Clinical Nutritionist & Naturopathic Physician who has been serving others for over 30 years. Dr. Martin is the Director of NUTRITION WELLNESS CENTER, LLC, a complementary/alternative family health facility in Sarasota, Florida.

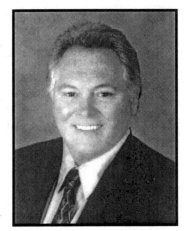

For decades Dr. Martin has lectured and devoted himself to researching the highest quality of nutritional alternatives. Dr. Martin dedicates his expertise solely to Nutrition, so that his knowledge and experience can reach more people in achieving their optimal health.

Dr. Martin has been featured on numerous television and radio programs and has had several nationally published articles. He has been noted as an expert in natural alternatives for achieving and maintaining wellness. Dr. Martin is a visionary leader of natural health whose expertise and experience has brought alternative medicine to a recognized level of helping people to reach their goals of optimal health and well-being.

Dr. Martin's Professional Affiliations Include:

- American Naturopathic Medical Association, *Board Certified*

- American Preventative Medical Association

- American Alternative Medical Association

- Florida Association of Naturopathic Medicine

- Fellow Status in the American Association of Integrative Medicine, *the highest honor awarded by the A.A.I.M.*

- Licensed Naturopath in Washington, D.C.

- Diplomat of the American Clinical Board of Nutrition, *the 1ˢᵗ & only organization in the United States that certifies professionals in nutrition that hold the distinction of accreditation*

Dr. Martin has been a Featured Guest Speaker to:

- **ABC-TV** Channel 7, with Health Newscaster Heidi Godman on "Nutrition & Children's Health"

- A seminar for **Health Professionals** at two **Annual Nutritional Symposiums**, Ogden Utah, one year on "Heavy Metals" & the next year on "Multiple Sclerosis & Nutrition Topics"

- **Blake Hospital**, Bradenton, Florida, to the Pediatric Therapy Department's Speech Therapists, Occupational Therapists & Physical Therapists

- **The National Health Federation**

- **Healthbeat of America with Rochelle,** 1220AM talk radio, a nationally-syndicated radio show

- **Barnes & Noble Bookstore,** Sarasota, Florida, on <u>Eat Right for Your Type,</u> by Dr. Peter D'Adamo

- Community Service Lectures, to students in the Sarasota County Schools

Publishing Credits

Dr. James H. Martin, N.M.D., D.C.C.N., D.A.C.B.N., F.A.A.I.M., has been published in:

- **"The International Journal of Biosocial Research,"** with Dr. John Nash Ott

- **"Heart Health & Nutrition, a Cardiologist's Guide to Total Wellness,"** by Dr. Steven Sinatra, M.D., who chose Dr. Martin as one of "America's Healing All-Stars"

- **"Behavioral Kinesiology Newsletter,"** by Dr. John Diamond, M.D.

- **"Take Control of Your Health,"** newsletter by Dr. Joseph Mercola, M.D.

- **"Total Health"** national magazine

- **"Health and Wellness Magazine,"** Nashville, Tennessee

- **"Natural Awakenings Magazine,"** Sarasota, Florida

- **"Positive Change Magazine,"** Sarasota, Florida

BIBLIOGRAPHY

The following list of references is not a complete list of the numerous resources that were available to the author on the topic of toxins and alternative medicine. These references are notable and are a source of expertise and are recommended for further reading.

Baillie-Hamilton, Paula. <u>Toxic Overload.</u> New York, N.Y.: Penguin Publishers, 2005.

Baker, Sherry, Adams, Mike. "Research Links Plastics Containing Bisphenol A to Heart Disease and Diabetes" www.naturalnews.com/024207_BPA_health_plastics.html

Berkson, Lindsey. <u>Hormone Deception</u>: How Everyday Foods and Products are Disrupting Your Hormones, and How to Protect Yourself and Your Family. Lincolnwood, IL: Contemporary Books, 2000.

Berthold-Bond, Annie. <u>Better Basics for the Home: Simple Solutions for Less Toxic Living</u>. New York, NY: Three Rivers Press, 1999.

Berthold-Bond, Annie. <u>Clean and Green</u>. Woodstock, NY: Ceres Press, 1994.

Blaylock, Russell L. <u>Excitotoxins: The Taste That Kills.</u> Santa Fe, NM: Health Press, 1997.

Blaylock, Russell L. Health and Nutrition Secrets. Albuquerque, NM: Health Press, 2006.

Brott, Armin A., Lombard, Jay, and Renna, Christian. Balance Your Brain, Balance Your Life. Hoboken, NJ: John Willey & Sons, Inc., 2004.

Buist, Robert, PhD. Food Chemical Sensitivity. Garden City Park, New York: Avery Publishing Group, 1986.

Casdroph, Dr. H. Richard & Walker, Dr. Morton. Toxic Metal Syndrome. Garden City Park, N.Y.: Avery Publishing Group, 1995.

Challkem, Jack. The Inflammation Syndrome. New Jersey: Wiley & Sons, 2003.

Colbert, Don, M.D. Toxic Relief. Lake Mary, Florida: Siloam Press, 2001.

Colbert, Don, M.D. What You Don't Know May be Killing You. Lake Mary, Florida: Siloam Press, 2000.

Colborn, Theo, Dumanoski, Dianne & Myers, John Peterson. Our Stolen Future. New York, N.Y. : Penguin Group, 1997.

Davies, Kent and Wiles, Richard. "Pesticides in Baby Food" Environmental Working Group

Farrier, Daniel F. MD. & McClure, Mark J. DDS, FAGD, co –editors. "The Journal of Capital University of Integrative Medicine" Washington, DC: Volume 1, Number 1, 2001

Fife, Bruce, N.D. The Detox Book. Colorado: Health Wise, 2001.

Fitzgerald, Randall. The Hundred Year Lie. New York, N.Y.: Dutton Publishers, 2006.

Ginsberg, Dr. Gary & Toal, Brian. What' Toxic, What's Not? New York, N.Y.: Berkley Books, 2006.

Harte, John, Holdren, Cheryl, Schneider, Richard & Shirley, Christine. Toxics A to Z. Berkeley: University of California Press, 1991.

IAACN (The International and American Associations of Clinical Nutritionists) 2003 Symposium, "Nutrition & Cancer: Prevention, Assessment, and Support". Addison, Texas: IAACN, 2003.

Kaufman, Doug A. The Fungus Link. Rockwall, Texas: Media Trition, 2000.

Moses, Marion. Designer Poisons. San Francisco, Ca: Pesticide Education Center, 1995.

Overman, Dr. James, ND. Overcoming Parasites Naturally. Millersburg, Ohio: Overman's Healthy Choices, Inc., 2003.

Physicians for Social Responsibility, "Cancer and the Environment: What Healthcare Providers Should Know"

Randolph, Theron G., M.D...& Moss, Ralph W. An Alternative Approach to Allergies. New York: Harper & Row Publishers, 1990.

Rapp, Doris J. Our Toxic World: A Wake-Up Call. Penryn, CA: Personal Transformation Press, 2003.

Repetto, Robert, SB. Pesticides and the Immune System: The Public Health Risks. Washington, D.C.: The World Resource Institute, 1996.

Rogers, Sherry. Detoxify or Die. Sarasota, FL: Sand Key Company, Inc., 2002.

Rogers, Sherry. <u>Tired or Toxic?</u> Syracuse, NY: Prestige Publishers,, 2000

Schettler, Ted, M.D. M.P.H., Soloman, Gina,M.D., M.P.H., Valenti, Maria & Huddle, Annette, M.E.S. <u>Generations at Risk.</u> Cambridge, Massachusetts: MIT Press, 1999.

Shoemaker, Ritchie C. MD, Schaller, James MD, Schmidt, Patti. <u>Mold Warriors.</u> Baltimore, MD: Gateway Press, 2005.

Sustainable Cuisine White Papers (Earth Pledge Foundation)

Thornton, Joe. <u>Pandora's Poison.</u> Cambridge, Massachusetts: MIT Press, 2000.

Tenney, Louise. <u>Encyclopedia of Natural Remedies</u>. New York, NY: Gramercy Books, 2002.

Weintraub, Sky, ND. <u>The Parasite Menace</u>. UT: Woodland Publishing, 1998.

Whitaker, Julian. <u>Reversing Heart Disease: A Vital New Program to Help Prevent, Treat, and Eliminate Cardiac Problems Without Surgery</u>. New York, N.Y.: Warner Books, 2002.

Yiamouyiannis, Dr. John. <u>Fluoride, The Aging Factor.</u> Delaware, Ohio: Health Action Press, 1993.

CPSIA information can be obtained at www.ICGtesting.com
Printed in the USA
LVOW06s2103190715

446806LV00001B/1/P